P9-CFV-106

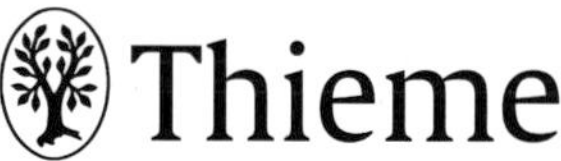
Thieme

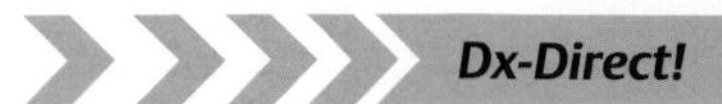
Dx-Direct!

Direct Diagnosis in Radiology

Urogenital Imaging

Bernd Hamm, MD
Professor and Chairman
Department of Radiology, Campus Mitte
Department of Radiotherapy, Campus Virchow-Klinikum
Charité – Universitätsmedizin Berlin
Berlin, Germany

Patrick Asbach, MD
Department of Radiology
Charité – Universitätsmedizin Berlin
Berlin, Germany

Dirk Beyersdorff, MD
Associate Professor
Department of Radiology
Charité – Universitätsmedizin Berlin
Berlin, Germany

Patrick Hein, MD
Department of Radiology
Charité – Universitätsmedizin Berlin
Berlin, Germany

Uta Lemke, MD
Department of Radiology
Charité – Universitätsmedizin Berlin
Berlin, Germany

233 Illustrations

Thieme
Stuttgart · New York

Library of Congress Cataloging-in-Publication Data

Urogenitales system. English.
Urogenital imaging / Bernd Hamm ... [et al.]; [translator, Bettina Herwig].
p. ; cm. – (Direct diagnosis in radiology)
Translation of: Urogenitales system / Bernd Hamm ... [et al.]. 2007.
Includes bibliographical references.
ISBN 978-3-13-145151-4 (alk. paper)
1. Genitourinary organs–Radiography–Handbooks, manuals, etc. I. Hamm, Bernd, Prof. Dr. II. Title. III. Series.
[DNLM: 1. Female Urogenital Diseases–radiography–Handbooks. 2. Male Urogenital Diseases–radiography–Handbooks. 3. Diagnosis, Differential–Handbooks. 4. Urography–Handbooks. WJ 39 U775 2008a]
RC874.U73513 2008
616.6'07572–dc22

2008002212

This book is an authorized and revised translation of the German edition published and copyrighted 2007 by Georg Thieme Verlag, Stuttgart, Germany. Title of the German edition: Pareto-Reihe Radiologie: Urogenitales System.

Translator: Bettina Herwig, Berlin, Germany

Illustrator: Markus Voll, Munich, Germany

Rüdigerstrasse 14, 70469 Stuttgart, Germany
http://www.thieme.de
Thieme New York, 333 Seventh Avenue, New York, NY 10001, USA
http://www.thieme.com

Cover design: Thieme Publishing Group
Typesetting by Ziegler + Müller, Kirchentellinsfurt, Germany
Printed by APPL, aprinta Druck, Wemding, Germany

ISBN 978-3-13-145151-4
(TPS, Rest of World)

1 2 3 4 5 6

Important note: Medicine is an ever-changing science undergoing continual development. Research and clinical experience are continually expanding our knowledge, in particular our knowledge of proper treatment and drug therapy. Insofar as this book mentions any dosage or application, readers may rest assured that the authors, editors, and publishers have made every effort to ensure that such references are in accordance with **the state of knowledge at the time of production of the book.**

Nevertheless, this does not involve, imply, or express any guarantee or responsibility on the part of the publishers in respect to any dosage instructions and forms of applications stated in the book. **Every user is requested to examine carefully** the manufacturers' leaflets accompanying each drug and to check, if necessary in consultation with a physician or specialist, whether the dosage schedules mentioned therein or the contraindications stated by the manufacturers differ from the statements made in the present book. Such examination is particularly important with drugs that are either rarely used or have been newly released on the market. Every dosage schedule or every form of application used is entirely at the user's own risk and responsibility. The authors and publishers request every user to report to the publishers any discrepancies or inaccuracies noticed. If errors in this work are found after publication, errata will be posted at www.thieme.com on the product description page.

1 Kidneys and Adrenals

P. Hein, U. Lemke, P. Asbach

2 The Urinary Tract

P. Asbach, D. Beyersdorff

3 *The Male Genitals*

U. Lemke, D. Beyersdorff, P. Asbach

4 *The Female Genitals*

U. Lemke, D. Beyersdorff, P. Asbach

3D Three-dimensional
ACKD Acquired cystic kidney disease
ACTH Adrenocorticotropic hormone
ADPKD Autosomal dominant polycystic kidney disease
ARPKD Autosomal recessive polycystic kidney disease
BPH Benign prostatic hyperplasia
bSSFP Balanced steady-state free precession
CIN Cervical intraepithelial neoplasia
CMV Cytomegalovirus
CNS Central nervous system
CT Computed tomography
CTA CT angiography
CTU CT urography
DTPA Diethylene triamine pentaacetic acid
EPO Erythropoietin
ESWL Extracorporeal shock wave lithotripsy
FDG Fluoro-18-deoxyglucose
FIGO Fédération Internationale de Gynécologie et d'Obstetrique
FSH Follicle-stimulating hormone
GnRH Gonadotropin-releasing hormone
GRE Gradient echo
HIV Human immunodeficiency virus
HLA Human leukocyte antigen
HNPCC Hereditary nonpolyposis colorectal cancer
HPV Human papilloma virus
HU Hounsfield unit
IR Inversion recovery
IVP Intravenous pyelogram
KUB Kidneys, ureters, and bladder
LH Luteinizing hormone
MEN Multiple endocrine neoplasia
MHC Major histocompatibility complex
MIP Maximum intensity projection
MPR Multiplanar reconstruction
MRA Magnetic resonance angiography
MRI Magnetic resonance imaging/image
NHL Non-Hodgkin lymphoma
PCR Polymerase chain reaction
PD Proton density
PET Positron emission tomography
PI Pulsatility index
PSA Prostate-specific antigen
PTA Percutaneous transluminal angioplasty
PTH Parathormone
RAS Renal artery stenosis
RCC Renal cell carcinoma
RI Resistance index
SE Spin echo
SIL Squamous intraepithelial lesion
TIRM Turbo inversion recovery magnitude
TRAS Transplant renal artery stenosis
TSE Turbo spin echo
TURB/TURBT Transurethral resection of bladder tumor
TURP Transurethral resection of the prostate
UAE Uterine artery embolization
UPJ Ureteropelvic junction
UTI Urinary tract infection
UVJ Ureterovesical junction

VCUG	Voiding cystourethrogram
VIN	Vulvar intraepithelial neoplasia
VUR	Vesicoureteral reflux

Definition

- **Etiology**

  Renal ectopia: During embryogenesis the developing kidneys ascend from the true pelvis into the lumbar region • Failure to ascend results in renal ectopia, pelvic kidney being the most common form • Less common are lumbosacral or thoracic kidneys and crossed renal ectopia with asymmetric fusion of the two kidneys on the same side of the body.

  Malrotation: Common • Anteriorly, laterally, or posteriorly directed renal pelvis.

  Duplex kidney: Kidney with two separate pelvicaliceal systems connected by a column of renal parenchyma.

  Horseshoe kidney: Kidneys fused at lower pole • Ascent arrested by inferior mesenteric artery • Kidneys connected by a parenchymal or fibrous isthmus • Typically associated with ureteropelvic junction obstruction, ureteral duplication, and genital tract anomalies.

Imaging Signs

- **Modality of choice**

  IVP • Ultrasound • CT • MRI.
- **Intravenous pyelogram findings**
  - *Ectopic/horseshoe kidney:* Location, shape.
  - *Duplex kidney:* Two renal pelves that drain separately.
- **Ultrasound, CT, and MRI findings**
  - *Pelvic kidney:* Renal artery supplying the kidney arises from the aorta at a lower level or from the ipsilateral iliac artery.
  - *Horseshoe kidney:* Mediolaterally directed parenchyma • Medial position of lower calices • Renal pelves face anteriorly • Isthmus located anterior to the abdominal aorta and inferior vena cava and posterior to the inferior mesenteric artery • Evaluation of vascular anatomy by CT after intravenous contrast administration.
  - *Duplex kidney:* Parenchymal isthmus between separate collecting systems.
  - *Malrotation:* Usually detected incidentally.

Clinical Aspects

- **Typical presentation**
  - Usually an incidental finding.
  - *Horseshoe/pelvic kidney:* May be complicated by obstruction, infection, or calculus formation.
  - Increased risk of injury in trauma.
  - Some patients may present with secondary hypertension due to stenosis of an accessory renal artery/polar artery.
- **Treatment options**

  Symptomatic treatment.

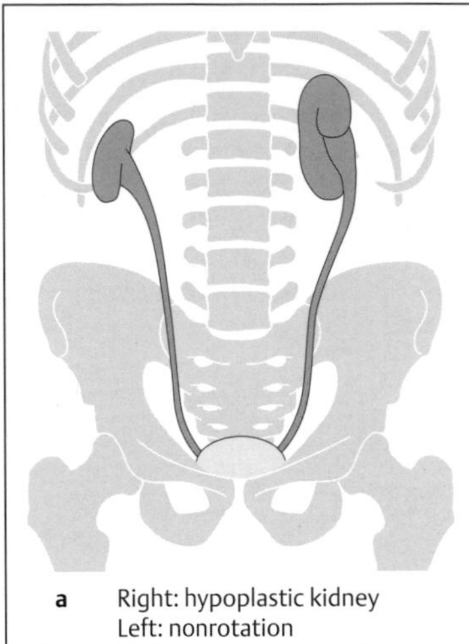

a Right: hypoplastic kidney
Left: nonrotation

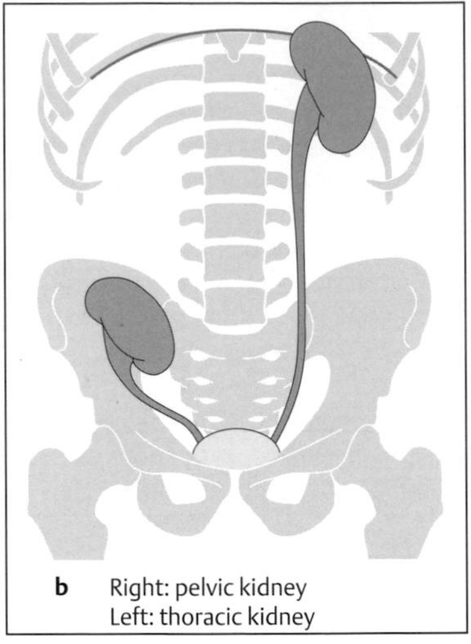

b Right: pelvic kidney
Left: thoracic kidney

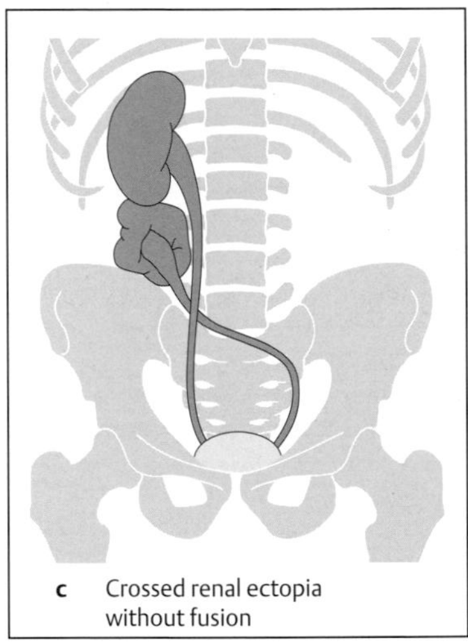

c Crossed renal ectopia
without fusion

Fig. 1.1 a–c Diagrammatic representation of major renal anomalies.

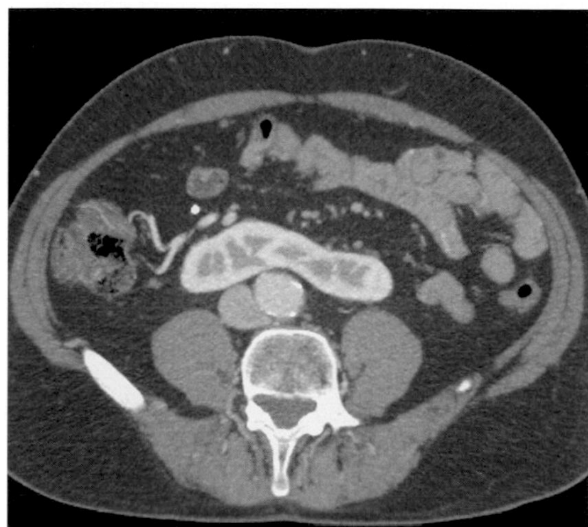

Fig. 1.2 Horseshoe kidney. Axial MPR from contrast-enhanced multislice CT. Preaortic parenchymal isthmus of the horseshoe kidney. The fused kidney is just below the inferior mesenteric artery.

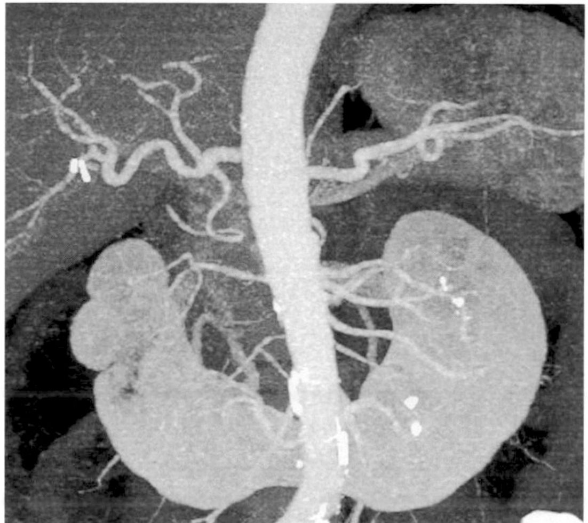

Fig. 1.3 Horseshoe kidney. Coronal MIP reconstruction.

- **Course and prognosis**
  Good prognosis if there are no complications.
- **What does the clinician want to know?**
  Diagnosis • Exact location • Presence of complications.

Differential Diagnosis

Nephroptosis (floating/wandering kidney)	– Downward displacement of the kidney; acquired condition characterized by excessive descent of the kidney when the body is erect – Differs from pelvic kidney in that the paired renal arteries are found in their typical locations – If additional rotation occurs, there is the risk of vascular compression/torsion or ureteral compression with intermittent hydronephrosis
Duplicated renal pelvis	– Usually one renal pelvis drains the upper group of calices and a second drains the middle and lower groups – The two renal pelves unite proximally

Tips and Pitfalls

Parenchymal isthmus of a horseshoe kidney can be misdiagnosed as a preaortic lymphoma on ultrasound.

Selected References

Cocheteux B et al. Rare variations in renal anatomy and blood supply: CT appearances and embryological background. A pictorial essay. Eur Radiol 2001; 11: 779–786

Definition

A developmental abnormality characterized by cystic dilatation of the collecting tubules in the medullary pyramids. *Synonyms:* Renal tubular ectasia and Cacchi–Ricci disease.

- **Epidemiology, etiology**
  Prevalence: 5:10 000 to 5:100 000 • More commonly affects both kidneys • Rarely familial • Associated with Beckwith–Wiedemann syndrome, Ehlers–Danlos syndrome, hyperparathyroidism, and congenital pyloric stenosis • Etiology unknown.

Imaging Signs

- **Modality of choice**
  IVP, contrast-enhanced CT (CT IVP).
- **Radiographic findings (abdominal plain film—KUB)**
  Plain radiograph may be normal or show nephrocalcinosis/nephrolithiasis.
- **Intravenous pyelogram findings**
  - Linear densities in the renal pyramids due to ectatic tubules/cystic cavities • Restricted to the papillary portion of the pyramids.
  - "Paintbrush" appearance due to the presence of contrast within dilated collecting ducts (Bellini ducts) in the medullary pyramids.
  - *Mild ductal ectasia:* Linear striations.
  - *Moderate ductal ectasia:* Grapelike clusters of rounded cystic opacities in the papillae, enlarged papillae, splaying of the caliceal cups.
  - *Severe disease:* Gross cystic changes with marked distortion of the calices.
  - Hydronephrosis in the presence of obstruction.
- **CT findings**
  - Unenhanced CT: Normal-sized, large, or small kidney • Cortical depressions in the presence of scars • Multiple calcifications visible with complications such as nephrocalcinosis or nephrolithiasis • Hydronephrosis in patients with obstruction.
  - CT after intravenous contrast administration, CT IVP: "Paintbrush" appearance and same degrees of severity as with IVP (see "Intravenous pyelogram findings" above) • Nephrocalcinosis/nephrolithiasis • Determination of the site of obstruction in patients with obstructive complications.
- **Ultrasound findings**
  Pyramidal calcifications identified as hyperechoic foci with acoustic shadowing • Cystic lesions.

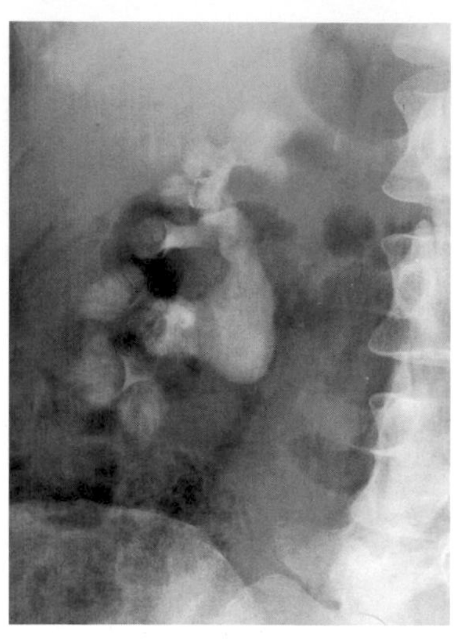

Fig. 1.4 Medullary sponge kidney. IVP 20 minutes after contrast infusion. Marked tubular ectasia.

Clinical Aspects

- **Typical presentation**
  - Asymptomatic in the absence of complications.
  - *Complications:* Hypercalciuria • Nephrolithiasis • Nephrocalcinosis.
  - *Clinical presentations associated with complications:* Urolithiasis • Recurrent hematuria • Urinary tract infections • Reduced maximal urinary concentrating ability • Incomplete distal tubular acidosis.
- **Treatment options**
  Symptomatic treatment: Thiazides, antibiotics, ESWL.
- **Course and prognosis**
  Depend on complications.
- **What does the clinician want to know?**
  Diagnosis • Detection of nephrocalcinosis/nephrolithiasis • Detection and location of calculi • Presence of obstruction.

Differential Diagnosis

Renal papillary necrosis	– Clinical presentation
Renal tuberculosis	– Clinical presentation, pathogen detection
Papillary blush	– Normal finding on IVP associated with contrast dose
Distal renal tubular acidosis	– In the presence of nephrocalcinosis
Primary hyperparathyroidism	– In the presence of nephrocalcinosis

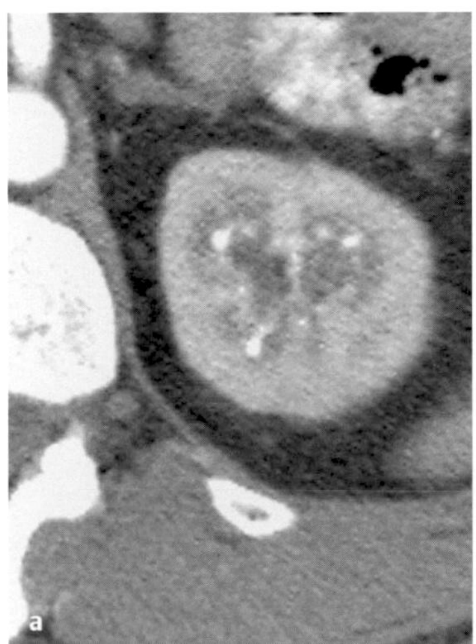

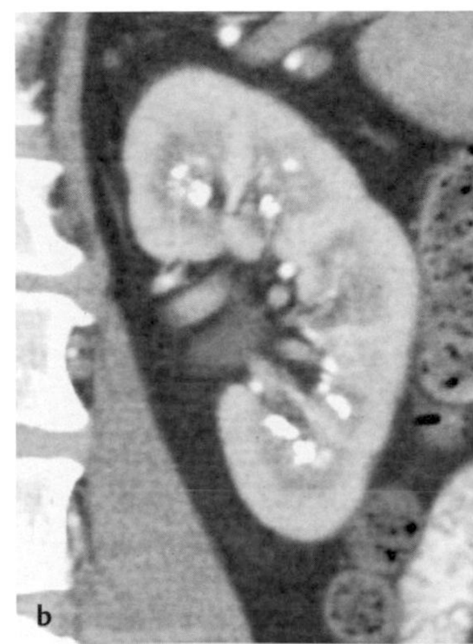

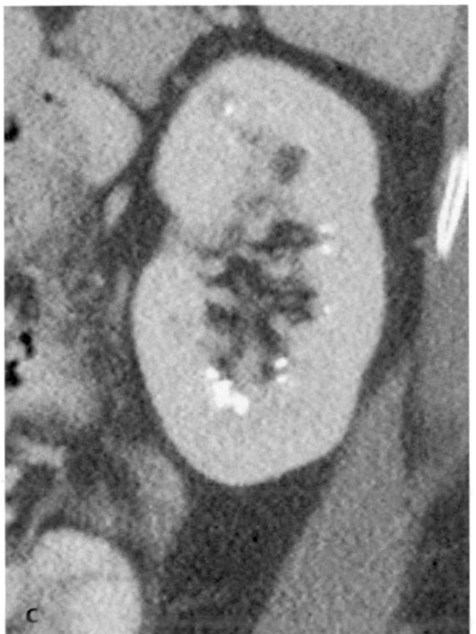

Fig. 1.5 a–c Medullary sponge kidney. Multiple, partially striated, calcifications. No obstruction.

- **a** Postcontrast axial multislice CT in the cortical phase.
- **b** Coronal MPR from the cortical phase.
- **c** Coronal MPR from the corticomedullary phase.

Selected References

Patriquin HB, O'Regan S. Medullary sponge kidney in childhood. AJR 1985; 145: 315–319
Thomsen HS et al. Renal cystic disease. Eur Radiol 1997; 7: 1267–1275

Definition

- **Epidemiology**
  Common anatomic variant.
- **Etiology**
  Accessory renal arteries may occur as polar arteries or as arteries entering the renal hilum.

Imaging Signs

- **Modality of choice**
  CTA • MRA.
- **CT and MRI technique**
  Contrast bolus timing by means of bolus tracking or test bolus injection for optimal arterial phase imaging • Acquisition of a 3D data set.

Clinical Aspects

- **Typical presentation**
  Usually asymptomatic • Some patients may present with renovascular hypertension due to accessory renal artery stenosis.
- **Treatment options**
  Treatment only in symptomatic patients.
- **What does the clinician want to know?**
  Diagnosis • Preoperative assessment of vascular anatomy in living kidney donors.

Tips and Pitfalls

Thin-slice data set acquired by multislice spiral CT or MRA is necessary to identify tiny accessory renal arteries.

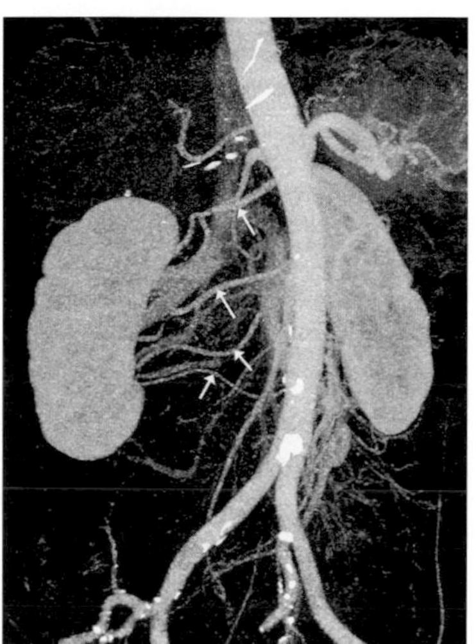

Fig. 1.6 Multiple arteries supplying the right kidney. MIP reconstruction from contrast-enhanced multislice CT data. The individual renal arteries are indicated by arrows.

Definition

Luminal narrowing of the renal artery.

▸ **Epidemiology, etiology**

Atherosclerosis: Most common cause of RAS • Luminal narrowing due to atherosclerotic plaque with/without calcification. Plaque may have fibrotic/soft components • More common in men • Bilateral RAS in 30–40% of cases • Atherosclerotic RAS typically at the origin of the renal artery from the abdominal aorta.
Fibromuscular dysplasia: Second most common cause • Noninflammatory fibrotic thickening of the vessel wall • Typically caused by medial fibroplasia, less frequently by intimal or periarterial fibroplasia • Bilateral in two thirds of cases • More common in women • Lesions usually affect the middle or distal segment of the renal artery • No calcinosis of the vessel wall.
Rare causes: Aortic dissection/aneurysm • Takayasu arteritis • Polyarteritis nodosa • Neurofibromatosis • Retroperitoneal fibrosis • Irradiation • Thromboembolism • Tumor compression.

Imaging Signs

▸ **Modality of choice**

Color Doppler ultrasound • CTA • MRA.

▸ **Ultrasound findings**

Peak systolic velocity ≥ 190 cm/s and RI < 0.55 indicate hemodynamically significant RAS • Turbulent flow in the poststenotic segment • Tardus/parvus waveform with delayed acceleration and rounded systolic peak distal to the stenosis.

▸ **CT findings**

Unenhanced CT to detect calcified plaques in the renal artery • High spatial resolution and optimal bolus timing/opacification are important for CTA • CT tends to overestimate stenosis.
Atherosclerosis: Concentric/eccentric stenosis • Focal or segmental ostial stenosis • Poststenotic dilatation may be present • Identification of plaque • Use of an automated vessel analysis tool can be helpful.
Fibromuscular dysplasia: Characteristic string-of-beads appearance of the artery with segmental stenoses • Circumscribed dilatations/aneurysms • Cortical/corticomedullary phase images will show delayed parenchymal enhancement, delayed excretion, and infarction.

▸ **MRI findings**

T1-weighted 3D GRE sequence after intravenous contrast administration for MPR or MIP reconstruction • Findings as on CTA.

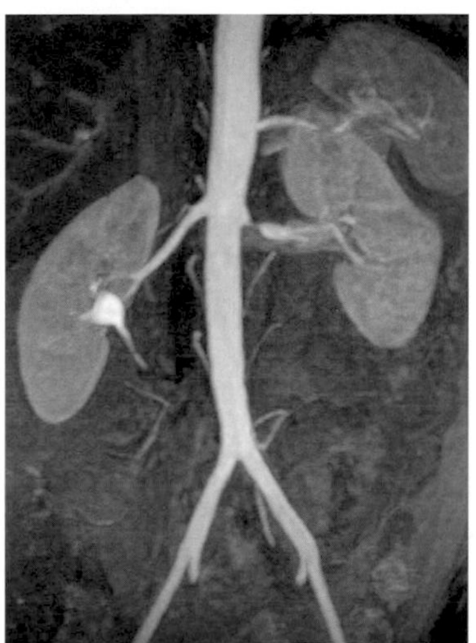

Fig. 1.7 Renal artery stenosis. Coronal MIP from MRA data. Atherosclerotic RAS near the origin of the left renal artery.

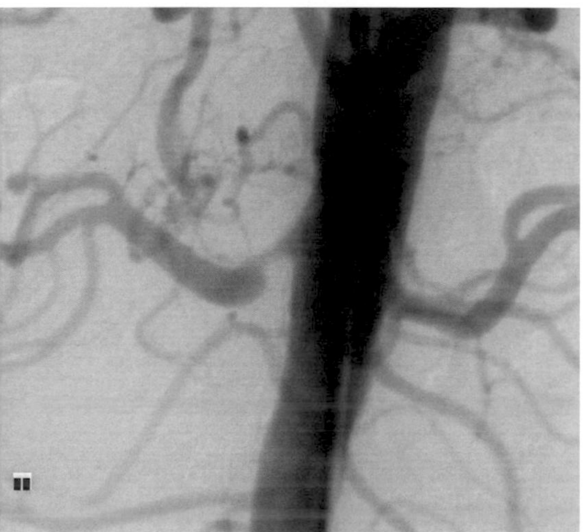

Fig. 1.8 Angiogram. Atherosclerotic stenosis of the right renal artery.

Clinical Aspects

- **Typical presentation**
  Secondary arterial hypertension with very high blood pressure • Renovascular hypertension in children or young adults suggests fibromuscular dysplasia • Renovascular hypertension in adults suggests atherosclerosis • Partial or complete loss of renal function • Systolic/diastolic bruit over the flank.
  Complications: thrombosis, dissection with renal artery occlusion and renal infarction, pulmonary edema and left ventricular decompensation in case of severe hypertension.
- **Treatment options**
  Angioplasty • Vascular surgery • Antihypertensive therapy.
- **Follow-up after treatment**
  CTA for follow-up after stenting (stent produces signal void on MRA).
- **What does the clinician want to know?**
  Hemodynamic relevance • Parenchymal damage • Interventional therapy possible?

Tips and Pitfalls

Renal artery stenosis may be overlooked if the CT/MRI slices are too thick • Proper timing is important for CTA/MRA.

Selected References

Herborn CU et al. Renal arteries: comparison of steady-state free precession MR angiography and contrast-enhanced MR angiography. Radiology 2006; 239: 263–268

Leiner T et al. Contemporary imaging techniques for the diagnosis of renal artery stenosis. Eur Radiol 2005; 15: 2219–2229

Definition

Ischemic necrosis of renal parenchyma • Focal or global • Acute, subacute or chronic.

▸ **Etiology, pathophysiology**

Causes:

Mainly caused by acute occlusion of an artery supplying the kidney due to:
- Thrombosis: Atherosclerosis • Polyarteritis nodosa • Conditions predisposing to thrombosis.
- Embolism: Atrial fibrillation • Endocarditis • Myocardial infarction • Catheter angiography.
- Trauma: Blunt abdominal trauma.

Anatomic extent:
- Subsegmental or segmental infarct (occlusion of a subsegmental/segmental artery) • One or more infarcted areas.
- Global infarct (occlusion of the main renal artery).
- Unilateral global infarct: Suggests thrombosis/trauma.
- Bilateral multiple (sub-)segmental infarcts: suggest embolism.

Imaging Signs

▸ **Modality of choice**

Ultrasound • CT • MRI.

▸ **General**

Extent of renal infarction can be assessed by contrast-enhanced CT/MRI or color Doppler ultrasound.

▸ **Ultrasound findings**

Color Doppler ultrasound demonstrates focal or complete absence of blood flow in the renal parenchyma • Can also be demonstrated by contrast-enhanced ultrasound.

▸ **CT findings**

Extent of infarcted area:
- Subsegmental: Sharply demarcated, wedge-shaped area of decreased enhancement • Wedge base at the renal capsule.
- Segmental: Sharply delineated • Due to occlusion of a segmental artery.
- Global: Complete absence of renal enhancement • No contrast excretion • "Spoke wheel" enhancement pattern is occasionally seen if there is collateral supply • Cortical rim sign indicates (sub-)capsular blood flow.

Acute versus chronic infarction:
- Acute: Normal-sized kidney with smooth contour • Reduced enhancement confined to a sharply demarcated area or throughout the kidney • No or reduced contrast excretion • Cortical rim sign.
- Chronic: Irregular renal contour • Small kidney due to parenchymal thinning • No cortical rim sign.

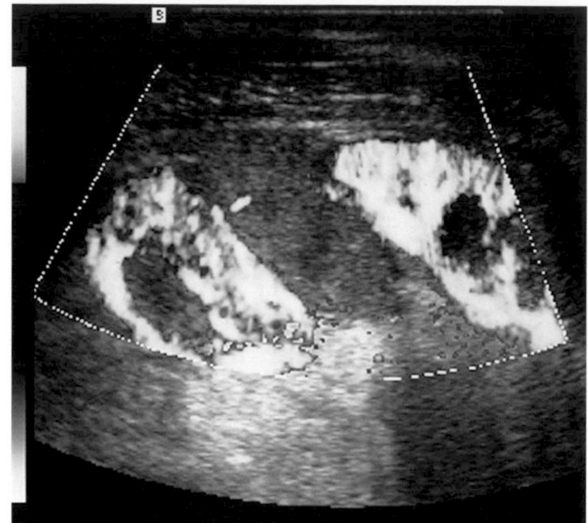

Fig. 1.9 Renal infarction. Color Doppler ultrasound showing perfusion defect in the middle third of the kidney.

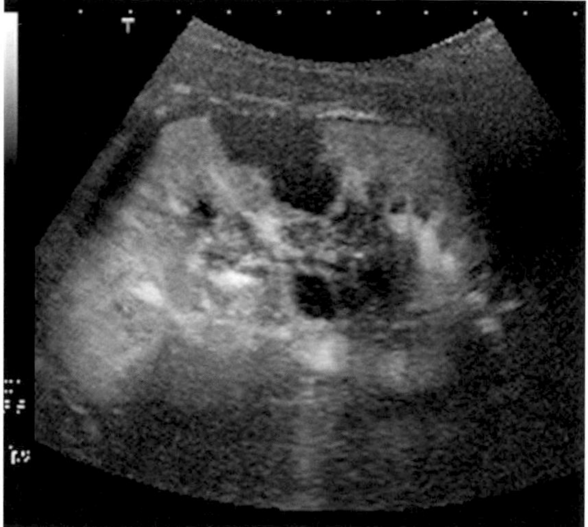

Fig. 1.10 Contrast-enhanced ultrasound. No uptake of contrast in the infarcted area.

- **Angiographic findings**
  Selective renal angiography • Identification of the site of vascular occlusion.
- **MRI findings**
  Older infarction isointense on T1-weighted images and hypointense on T2-weighted images • Parenchymal thinning • Findings on contrast-enhanced T1-weighted images similar to contrast-enhanced CT.

Clinical Aspects

- **Typical presentation**
  Flank pain • Hematuria • Hypertension • Chronic renal failure in some patients.
- **Treatment options**
  Anticoagulant therapy • Angioplasty with thrombolytic therapy in patients with fresh or incomplete arterial occlusion.
- **Course and prognosis**
  Depend on the extent of infarction, underlying cause, and presence of (late) complications.
- **What does the clinician want to know?**
  Confirmation of the diagnosis • Extent of infarction • Bilateral infarction?

Differential Diagnosis

Pyelonephritis	– Typically less sharply demarcated hypodensities/ hypointensities – No cortical rim sign – Clinical signs and symptoms
Lymphoma	– Lesion not wedge shaped

Selected References

Garovic VD, Textor SC. Renovascular hypertension and ischemic nephropathy. Circulation 2005; 112: 1362–1374

Suzer O et al. CT features of renal infarction. Eur J Radiol 2002; 44: 59–64

Definition

Thrombotic occlusion of one or both main renal veins.

- **Etiology**
  - *Causes in adults:* Tumor • Infection • Nephrotic syndrome • Post partum • Hypercoagulable state.
  - *Causes in children:* Shock • Trauma • Sepsis • Conditions predisposing to thrombosis such as sickle cell anemia.

Imaging Signs

- **Modality of choice**
  Ultrasound • CT • MRI.
- **Ultrasound findings**
  - *Acute:* Kidney enlarged • Color Doppler ultrasound depicts no flow in the renal vein • Vascular dilatation • Hypoechoic cortex due to acute edema with preserved corticomedullary differentiation.
  - *Chronic:* Small kidney with loss of corticomedullary differentiation • Hyperechoic parenchyma due to chronic degeneration (e.g., fibrosis).
- **CT findings**
  Hypodense thrombus (filling defect) in the renal vein, best appreciated in the corticomedullary phase (venous phase) after contrast administration • Vascular dilatation • Venous collaterals in chronic thrombosis • Renal pelvis may be compressed.
- **MRI findings**
  T1-weighted sequence after intravenous contrast administration • Thrombus seen as filling defect • Vascular dilatation.

Clinical Aspects

- **Typical presentation**
  Acute onset • Flank pain • Gross hematuria.
- **Treatment options**
  Heparin therapy • Anticoagulation therapy • Treatment of nephrotic syndrome.
- **What does the clinician want to know?**
  Extent • Parenchymal damage • Identification of underlying cause if present (e.g., tumor).

Differential Diagnosis

Tumor thrombus in RCC	– Contains enhancing tumor vessels

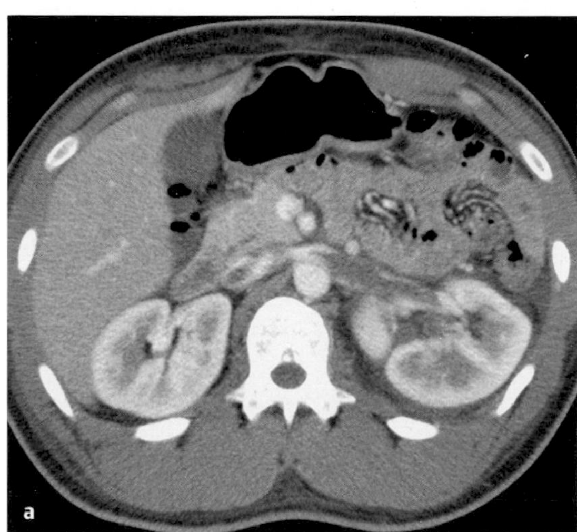

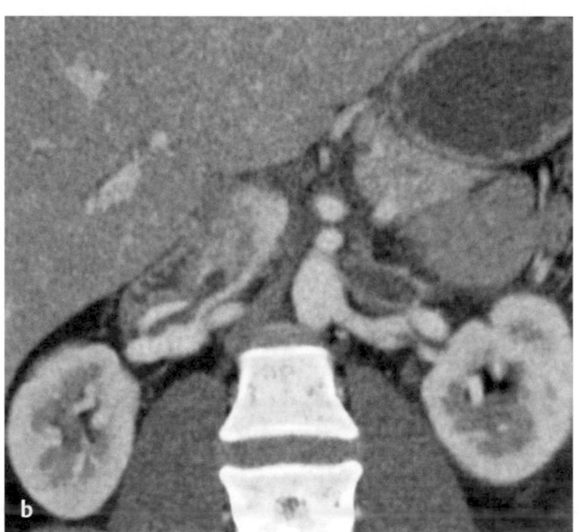

Fig. 1.11 a, b Postpartum bilateral renal vein thrombosis.

a Axial multislice CT scan after contrast administration. Dilated left renal vein with intraluminal filling defect.

b Coronal reconstruction showing the thrombus protruding from the right renal vein into the inferior vena cava.

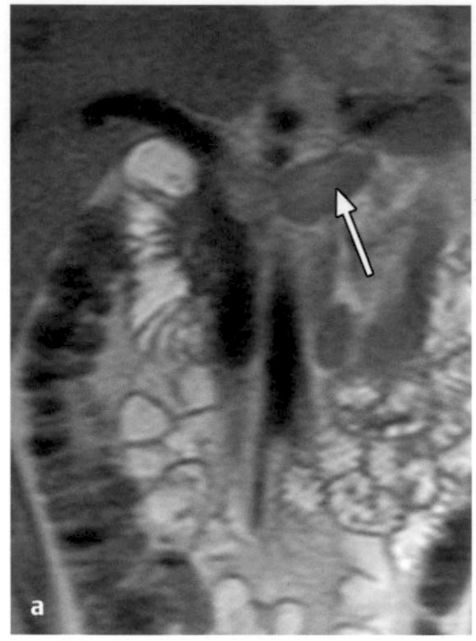

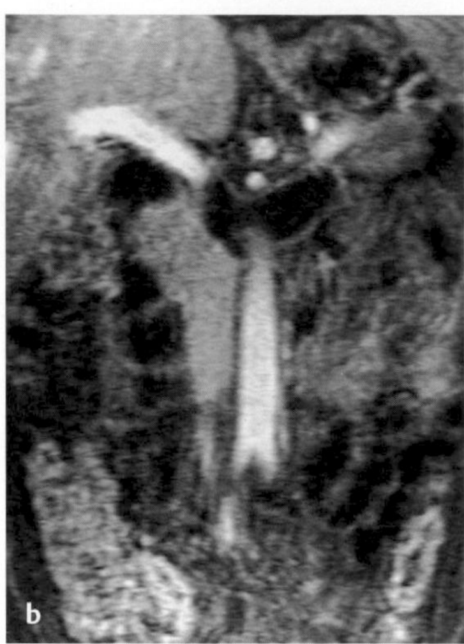

Fig. 1.12 a, b Thrombosis of the left renal vein. The thrombus dilates the left renal vein, which crosses in front of the aorta (arrow in **a**).
a Unenhanced coronal T2-weighted MR image.
b Fat-suppressed T1-weighted MR venography obtained in a comparable plane after intravenous administration of a nonspecific, gadolinium-based contrast medium.

Tips and Pitfalls

Do not acquire contrast-enhanced images before proper opacification of the veins has occurred.

Selected References

Kawashima A et al. CT evaluation of renovascular disease. Radiographics. 2000; 20: 1321–1340

Definition

- **Etiology**
  Predominant causes: blunt abdominal trauma, penetrating injuries, and iatrogenic trauma (interventional procedures, surgery).
  Classification according to severity and clinical symptoms:
  - *Minor lesions* (> 80% of cases): Intrarenal hematoma • Contusion • Small subcapsular laceration • Subcapsular hematoma • Small perinephric hematoma • Subsegmental infarction.
  - *Major lesions* (10%): Large cortical laceration • Large perinephric hematoma • Segmental infarction • Involvement of the renal sinus with extravasation of urine.
  - *Catastrophic injuries:* Multiple parenchymal lacerations • Vascular injury • Involvement of the renal pedicle.
  - *Injury to the ureteropelvic junction* (rare).

Imaging Signs

- **Modality of choice**
  CT to demonstrate hematoma, infarction, and injury to the collecting system.
- **Pathognomonic findings**
  Striated or wedge-shaped areas of reduced enhancement in the renal parenchyma • Swollen kidney.
- **CT findings**
  Unenhanced CT: Hyperdense or isodense hematoma • Rounded and irregular lesion indicates intrarenal contusion • Crescent-shaped lesion indicates subcapsular hematoma with intact capsule • Size of perirenal hematoma correlates with the extent of injury; its location corresponds to the site of parenchymal laceration.
  CT after intravenous contrast administration:
  - *Contusion:* Corticomedullary phase—rounded hypodensity in parenchyma • Urographic phase—hyperdense lesion due to contrast retention in parenchyma.
  - *Subcapsular or perinephric hematoma:* Corticomedullary phase—crescent or linear • Attenuation of 40–80 HU.
  - *Small laceration:* Corticomedullary phase—linear hypodensity • Located peripherally.
  - *Large laceration:* Corticomedullary phase—sharply demarcated, wedge-shaped hypodensity • Large perirenal hematoma.
  - *Concomitant rupture of the collecting system:* Corticomedullary phase—hypodense lesion extending into the renal sinus • Urographic phase—perirenal extravasation of contrast medium • Contrast excretion into the ureter may be absent.
  - *Multiple lacerations and vascular injuries:* Cortical and corticomedullary phases—several hypodense areas • Heterogeneous appearance of hematoma • Escape of contrast medium indicates active arterial bleeding.

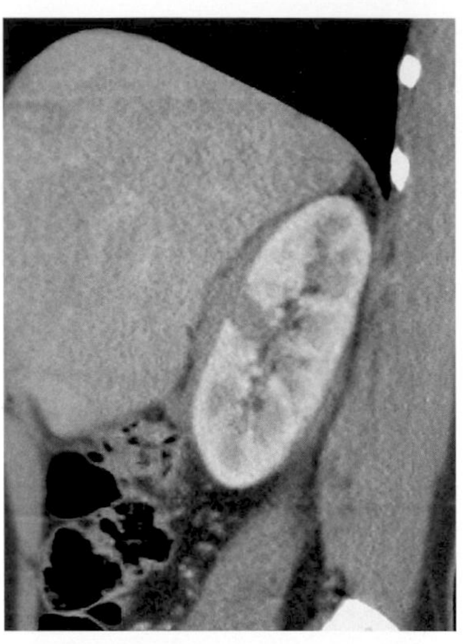

Fig. 1.13 Small focal contusion with minor capsular tear. Sagittal MPR from multislice CT after contrast administration in the cortical phase.

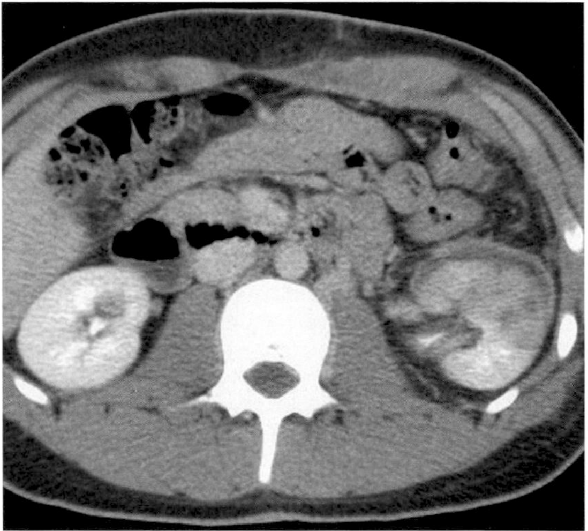

Fig. 1.14 Laceration with subcapsular hematoma. Axial image after contrast administration in the corticomedullary phase.

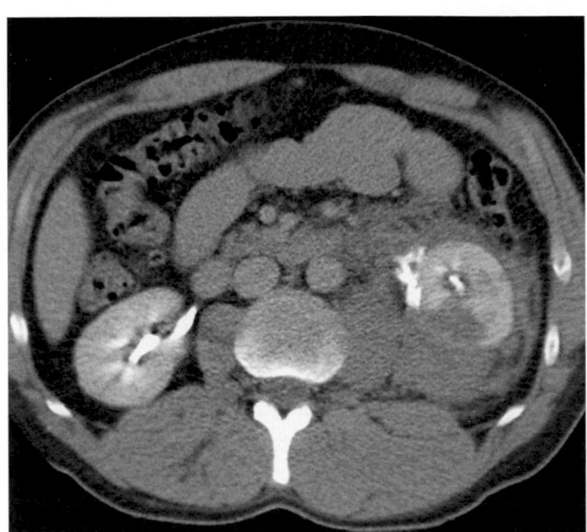

Fig. 1.15 Cortical laceration with perinephric hematoma. Axial contrast-enhanced CT scan in the urographic phase showing involvement of the renal pelvis.

- *Rupture of the ureteropelvic junction:* Cortical/corticomedullary phase—normal enhancement of renal parenchyma and normal contrast excretion • Urographic phase—perirenal urine leakage and opacified urinoma.
- *Subsegmental renal infarction:* Wedge shaped • Hypodense • Cortical.
- *Segmental renal infarction:* Reduced contrast accumulation in anterior/posterior aspect, upper/lower pole • Cortical rim sign.
- *Global renal infarction:* Secondary to renal artery avulsion or acute renal artery stenosis • Entire kidney is hypodense, indicating little or no perfusion.

Clinical Aspects

- **Typical presentation**

  Hematuria • Flank pain • Tenderness • Anemia • Shock • Involvement of other organs • Bone trauma.

  Complications: Uremia • Infection with abscess or sepsis • Possible formation of intramural arteriovenous fistula • Late sequelae include hypertension, chronic infection, and hydronephrosis.
- **Treatment options**
  - *Minor injury:* Conservative.
  - *Major injury:* Usually treated conservatively but occasionally requires surgery.
  - *Catastrophic injury:* Surgery.
  - *Active bleeding:* Interventional embolization.
  - *Renal artery thrombosis:* Anticoagulant treatment.
  - *Extravasation of urine:* Drainage, ureteral stent.

- **Course and prognosis**
  Depend on severity of injury and complications.
- **What does the clinician want to know?**
  Severity of renal injury • Involvement of the collecting system.

Tips and Pitfalls

Urinoma or rupture of the collecting system may be overlooked unless urographic phase images are obtained.

Selected References

Harris AC et al. CT findings in blunt renal trauma. Radiographics 2001; 21: 201–214

Kawashima A et al. Imaging of renal trauma: a comprehensive review. Radiographics 2001; 21: 557–574

Definition

An acute bacterial infection of the renal collecting system and parenchyma.

- **Epidemiology**
  Three times more common in women than men • Peak incidence during the first 3 years of life.
- **Etiology**
  Ascending UTI • Hematogenous spread (rare, occasionally in patients with sepsis) • Focal or diffuse • *Predisposing factors:* VUR, diabetes, pregnancy, immunocompromised status, urolithiasis • *Most common pathogen: Escherichia coli.*

Imaging Signs

- **Modality of choice**
  CT • MRI • Ultrasound (mainly for follow-up).
- **CT and MRI findings**
  Swollen and edematous kidney • Corticomedullary differentiation reduced or segmentally lost • Striated, segmental or wedge-shaped, areas of diminished enhancement on postcontrast CT or MRI • Increased contrast accumulation in the wall of the renal pelvis and ureter with induration of surrounding tissue • Perirenal fluid.
- **Ultrasound findings**
  Enlarged kidney • Inhomogeneous echotexture of renal parenchyma.
- **Intravenous pyelogram findings**
  Delayed and reduced opacification of the kidney • Caliceal effacement caused by swelling of adjacent parenchyma • Papillary necrosis in advanced disease.

Clinical Aspects

- **Typical presentation**
  Fever • Flank pain • Pyuria • Hematuria • Infants and children often present with nonspecific symptoms such as lethargy or poor general condition.
- **Treatment options**
  Antibiotic therapy • Adequate fluid intake • Abscess drainage • Causal therapy of predisposing conditions where possible.
- **Course and prognosis**
  Good prognosis in most patients • Poor prognosis in those rare cases where recurrent episodes lead to chronic pyelonephritis.
- **What does the clinician want to know?**
  Acute intervention (e.g., obstruction, abscess) necessary? • Predisposing conditions.

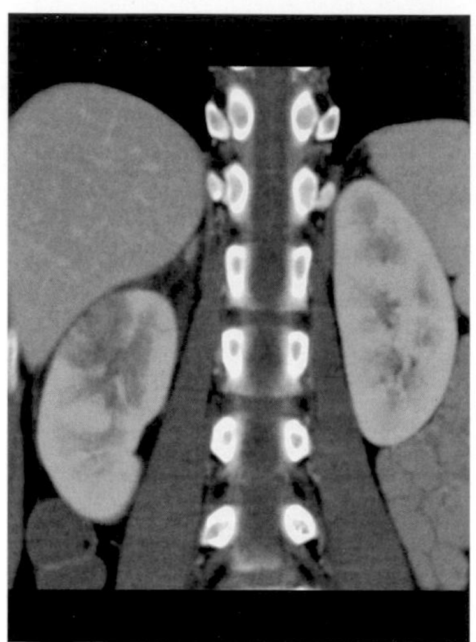

Fig. 1.16 Acute focal pyelonephritis of the right kidney. Coronal reconstruction from cortical phase CT data. Segmental area of reduced enhancement in the upper pole. Mild swelling of the upper third of the kidney.

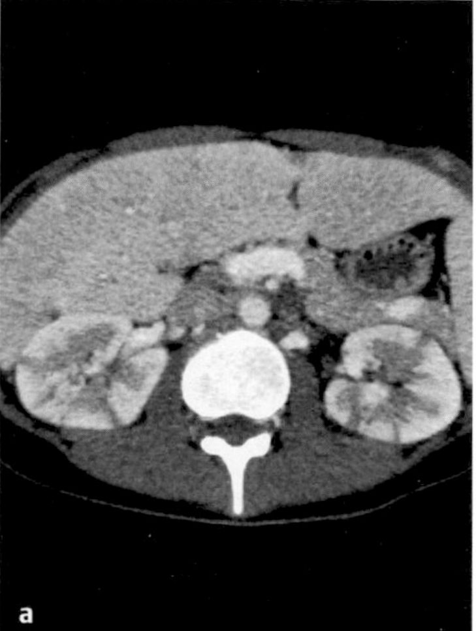

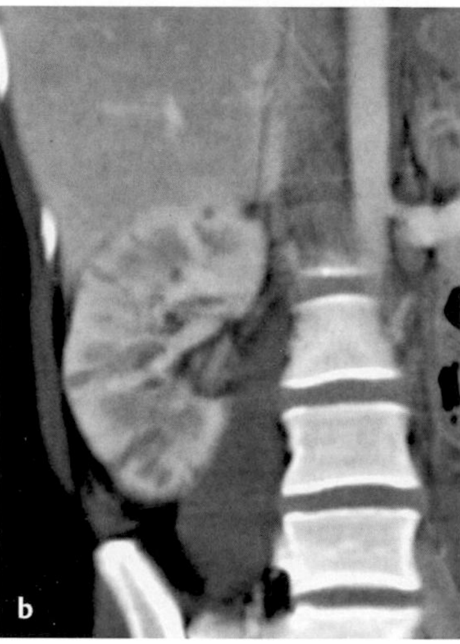

Fig. 1.17 a, b Acute diffuse pyelonephritis of both kidneys. Axial (**a**) and coronal (**b**) cortical phase CT scans. Multiple segmental areas of reduced perfusion in the renal cortex (striation).

Differential Diagnosis

Renal infarction	– Kidney not enlarged – Possible infarction of other organs (e.g., spleen)
Renal lymphoma	– Rounded lesions with reduced contrast enhancement – May be difficult to differentiate from focal acute pyelonephritis
Renal trauma	– History – Hematoma – Parenchymal laceration
Xanthogranulomatous pyelonephritis	– Parenchyma replaced by fibrotic scar tissue with fatty components (CT!)

Tips and Pitfalls

Do not misdiagnose pyelonephritis as a renal tumor • Carefully search for a possible underlying morphologic cause (anomaly).

Selected References

Bjerklund Johansen TE. The role of imaging in urinary tract infections. World J Urol 2004; 22: 392–398

Paterson A. Urinary tract infection: an update on imaging strategies. Eur Radiol 2004; 14: L89–L100

Ramakrishnan K, Scheid DC. Diagnosis and management of acute pyelonephritis in adults. Am Fam Physician 2005; 71: 933–942

Definition

Chronic interstitial renal infection with scar formation • Involves the collecting system and renal parenchyma • Must be differentiated from granulomatous pyelonephritis (xanthogranulomatous pyelonephritis and tuberculosis) • Primary pyelonephritis if no underlying cause is apparent • Secondary pyelonephritis if an underlying cause can be identified.

- **Epidemiology**
  More common in women than men • Peak incidence in childhood.
- **Etiology**
  Urinary obstruction • Reflux of infected urine (mainly in children) • Congenital anomalies • Most common route of infection is ascending UTI.

Imaging Signs

- **Modality of choice**
  CT • MRI.
- **Pathognomonic findings**
  Small kidney with parenchymal thinning • Cortical scarring.
- **CT and MRI findings**
  Loss of renal parenchyma due to scarring • Residual parenchyma accumulates contrast medium (though uptake may be reduced) • Caliceal dilatation • Thickening of the Gerota fascia • Perirenal fluid.
- **Ultrasound findings**
  Echodense renal cortex • Scars and parenchymal thinning • Caliceal dilatation.
- **Intravenous pyelogram findings**
  Small kidney • Evaluation of renal function, which may be reduced or completely lost • Caliceal clubbing • Dilated ureter • Calculi may be present.
- **Voiding cystourethrography findings**
  Diagnosis and grading of VUR.

Clinical Aspects

- **Typical presentation**
  Clinical symptoms are nonspecific • Dysuria • Weight loss • Poor general condition • Acute episode is associated with fever, flank pain, and pyuria.
- **Treatment options**
  Antibiotic treatment • Adequate fluid intake • Causal therapy if possible • Hemodialysis or kidney transplant in end-stage disease.
- **Course and prognosis**
  Good prognosis only if the diagnosis is timely and predisposing factors can be eliminated • Poor prognosis in advanced disease • End-stage disease: renal atrophy with complete loss of function.
- **What does the clinician want to know?**
  Underlying cause • Intrarenal and extrarenal extent of the inflammatory process.

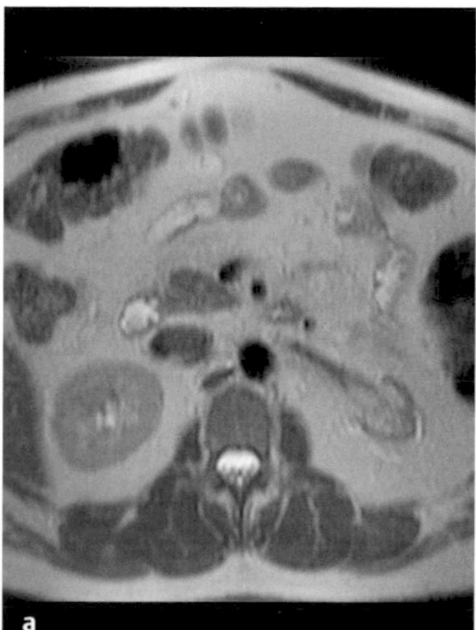

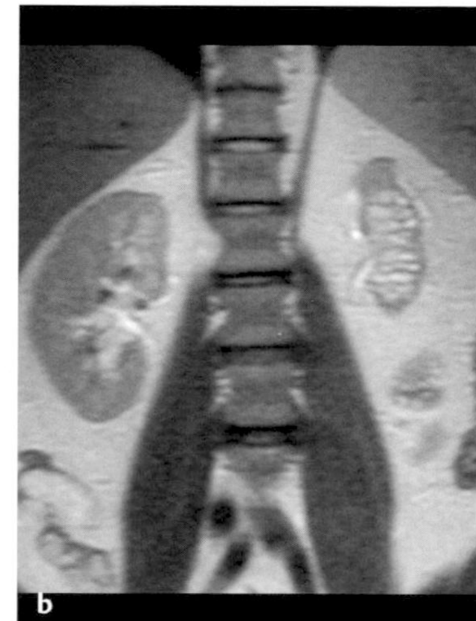

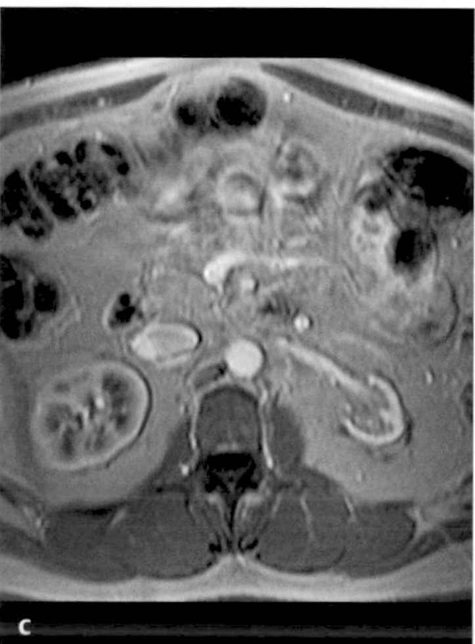

Fig. 1.18 a–c Atrophy of the left kidney as the end stage of chronic pyelonephritis. Marked loss of parenchyma with enhancement of the residual parenchyma. Small perirenal fluid collections.

- **a** Unenhanced axial T2-weighted single-shot TSE MR image.
- **b** Unenhanced coronal T2-weighted single-shot TSE MR image.
- **c** Contrast-enhanced axial T1-weighted GRE MR image.

Differential Diagnosis

Renal atrophy of vascular origin	– Markedly reduced or absent uptake of contrast medium by residual parenchyma
Renal hypoplasia	– No parenchymal scarring – Difficult to differentiate without considering clinical data
Granulomatous pyelonephritis	– Parenchyma replaced by fibrotic scar tissue – Presence of fat (xanthogranulomatous pyelonephritis) – Presence of calcifications (tuberculosis)
Hydronephrosis	– Marked distention of the pelvis and calices – May be associated with hydroureter

Tips and Pitfalls

Full evaluation of the renal pelvis, ureter, and bladder is necessary to identify the underlying cause.

Selected References

Bjerklund Johansen TE. The role of imaging in urinary tract infections. World J Urol 2004; 22: 392–398

Paterson A. Urinary tract infection: An update on imaging strategies. Eur Radiol 2004; 14: L89–L100

Definition

Uncommon renal interstitial disease characterized by parenchymal destruction developing secondary to chronic corticomedullary inflammation • Lymphocytic infiltrates with foam cells (lipid-laden macrophages) • Epithelioid cell granulomas.

- **Epidemiology**
  Very rare • Diffuse type (90%) • Focal type (10%).
- **Etiology**
  A chronic inflammatory reaction in the presence of large calculi or chronic ureteropelvic junction obstruction has been proposed • Chronic UTI.

Imaging Signs

- **Modality of choice**
  CT • MRI.
- **CT findings**
  CT after intravenous contrast administration: Obstructing pelvic or caliceal stone • Intraparenchymal calcifications • Kidney is enlarged but reniform shape is preserved • Multiple hypoattenuating masses (–15 to –30 HU) that do not enhance • Rim enhancement • Reduced urinary excretion of contrast medium • Inflammatory extension to perirenal tissue with fibrosis and thickening of the renal fascia.
- **MRI findings**
  T1-weighted image: hypointense areas • T2-weighted image: hyperintense areas • T1-weighted image after intravenous contrast administration: Lesions may show rim enhancement • Perirenal enhancement indicates extent of inflammatory process.

Clinical Aspects

- **Typical presentation**
  Very poor general condition • Fever • Flank pain • Reduced renal function • *Complications:* Sepsis, abscess.
- **Course and prognosis**
  Chronic inflammation • Confirmation of the diagnosis by biopsy.
- **Treatment options**
  Nephrectomy.
- **What does the clinician want to know?**
  Diagnosis • Exclusion of malignancy.

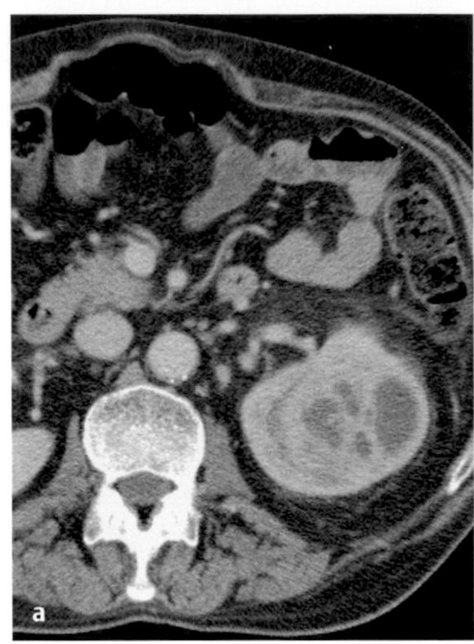

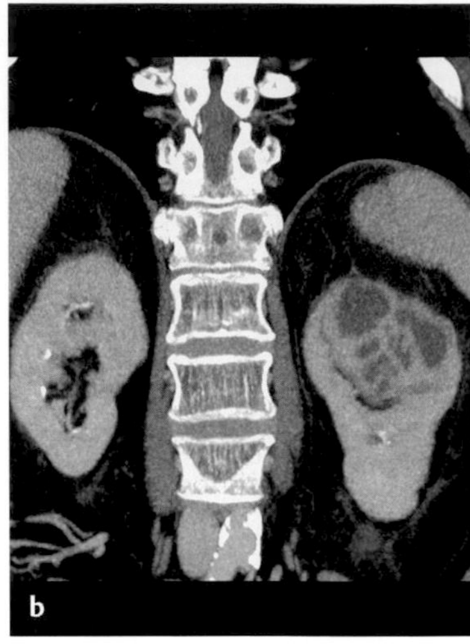

Fig. 1.19 a, b Xanthogranulomatous pyelonephritis of the left kidney.
a Axial CT scan in the corticomedullary phase. Marked enhancement of the residual parenchyma.
b Coronal MPR from the corticomedullary phase. There is increased attenuation of the renal fascia as a sign of perirenal inflammatory extension.

Differential Diagnosis

Pyonephrosis	– Distended pelvicaliceal system
RCC	– Rarely associated with calculi – Contrast enhancement
Renal lymphoma	– Rarely associated with calculi – Higher attenuation

Tips and Pitfalls

Do not misdiagnose xanthogranulomatous pyelonephritis as RCC.

Selected References

Hallscheidt P et al. Magnetic resonance tomography of xanthogranulomatous pyelonephritis. Epidemiology, pathogenesis and symptoms. Urologe A 2002; 41: 577–582

Verswijvel G et al. Xanthogranulomatous pyelonephritis: MRI findings in the diffuse and the focal type. Eur Radiol 2000; 10: 586–589

Definition

Distention of the renal pelvis and calices with pus.

- **Etiology**
  Urinary tract obstruction by calculi • Compression by mass • Anomaly • Postoperative strictures • Benign prostatic hyperplasia • Increased risk in patients with diabetes mellitus • Infection of dilated pelvicaliceal system.

Imaging Signs

- **Modality of choice**
  Ultrasound.
- **Ultrasound findings**
  Distention of pelvis and calices • Demonstration of pus • Echogenicity of the pelvicaliceal system differentiates pyonephrosis from uninfected hydronephrosis • Urine–pus level • Gas in the pelvis and ureter is identified by acoustic shadowing.
- **CT findings**
  CT is indicated only if ultrasound is not diagnostic • CT with intravenous contrast administration • Identification of the cause of pelvic and ureteral dilatation • Wall enhancement of the pelvicaliceal system • Attenuation values of 20–30 HU suggest pus or infected fluid • Sedimentation of cell debris • Multiphasic CT (CT IVP, may be performed in low-dose technique) will demonstrate absence of excretion (silent kidney).

Clinical Aspects

- **Typical presentation**
  Flank pain (dull) • Elevated temperature (low-grade fever to septicemic levels) • Pyuria • Raised levels of inflammatory markers.
- **Treatment options**
  Management of renal obstruction, e.g., by ureteral stent insertion • Antibiotic treatment.
- **Course and prognosis**
  Depend on the presence of complications • Can progress to necrosis and liquefaction, resulting in paranephric abscess • Urosepsis.
- **What does the clinician want to know?**
  Diagnosis • Cause of urinary obstruction.

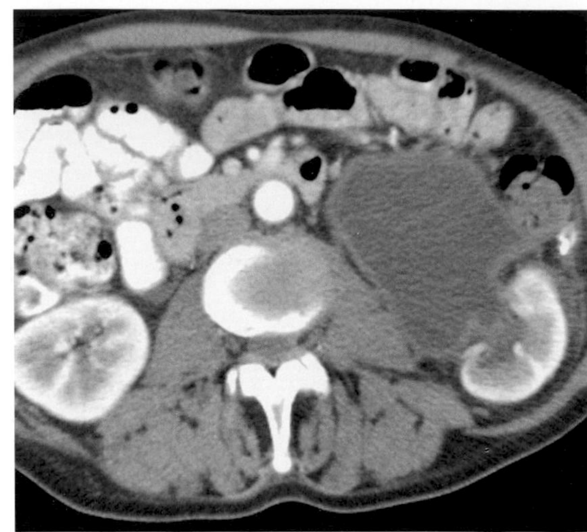

Fig. 1.20 Pyonephrosis of the left kidney. Axial multislice CT in the cortical phase. Distention of the renal pelvis and calices with wall enhancement. The fluid has an attenuation value of about 30 HU.

Differential Diagnosis

Pyelonephritis with abscess formation	– Differs from pyonephrosis in that the parenchyma appears patchy on contrast-enhanced CT scans – Hypodense areas, which may be wedge shaped, in the corticomedullary phase – Kidney may be swollen

Selected References

Browne RF et al. Imaging of urinary tract infection in the adult. Eur Radiol 2004; 14 (Suppl 3): E168–183

Paterson A. Urinary tract infection: an update on imaging strategies. Eur Radiol 2004; 14 (Suppl 4): L89–100

Definition

A localized collection of pus in the renal parenchyma • Called *renal carbuncle* when caused by confluent suppurative foci.

- **Epidemiology**
  Renal abscess accounts for 2% of all renal masses.
- **Etiology**
  Ascending UTI • Urolithiasis • Obstruction • Reflux • Urinary bladder catheter infection • Cystitis • Secondary to acute focal bacterial nephritis • Complication of pyelonephritis • Hematogenous spread in septicemia (*Staphylococcus aureus*, streptococci, enterococci) • Superinfection of a cyst or hematoma • *Predisposing conditions:* Diabetes mellitus, immunocompromised state (intravenous drug abuse, HIV).

Imaging Signs

- **Modality of choice**
  Ultrasound • Additional CT and/or MRI may be helpful.
- **Utrasound findings**
  Hypoechoic, rounded, thick-walled mass • Internal echoes from cell debris in the abscess change position when the patient is moved • Strong echoes with acoustic shadows indicate gas within the abscess.
- **CT findings**
  Unenhanced: Single or multiple lesions in one or both kidneys • Typically rounded and well-defined lesions of low attenuation • Reaction of surrounding tissue with increased attenuation of perirenal fat • Possible thickening of the Gerota fascia • Demonstration of gas.
  After intravenous contrast administration: Wall enhancement • No central enhancement • Attenuation value of 20–30 HU • Extensive abscess may distort and enlarge the renal contour • Renal sinus may be distorted or compressed • Distended pelvis with wall enhancement • May be septated/loculated • Smaller masses (microabscesses) are seen in the corticomedullary phase.
- **MRI findings**
  T1-weighted image: hypointense center • T2-weighted image: moderately hyperintense center • T1-weighted image after intravenous contrast administration: wall enhancement.
- **Intravenous pyelogram findings**
  Delayed and inhomogeneous nephrogram • One or more smoothly delineated, rounded lesions • Larger masses may distend the renal pelvis or cause splaying/effacement of calices.

Fig. 1.21 Multiple abscesses enlarging the right kidney. Cortical phase axial CT scan. The lesions are characterized by a hypodense center and peripheral enhancement.

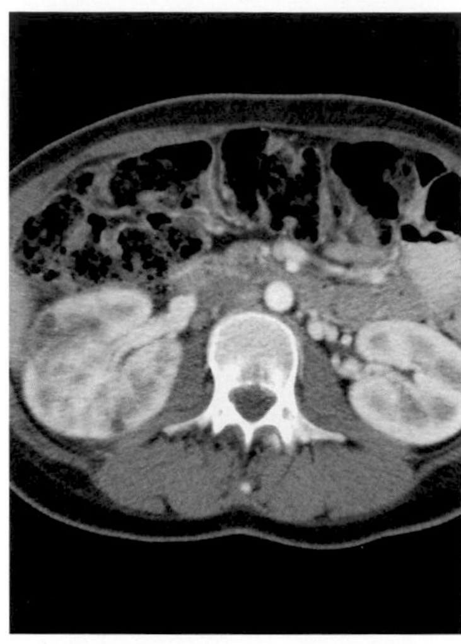

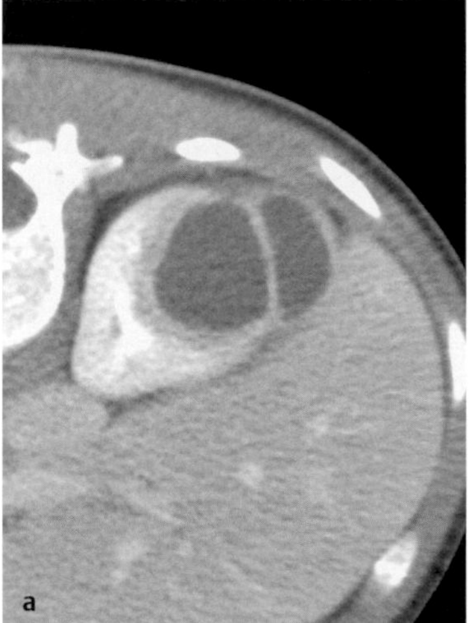

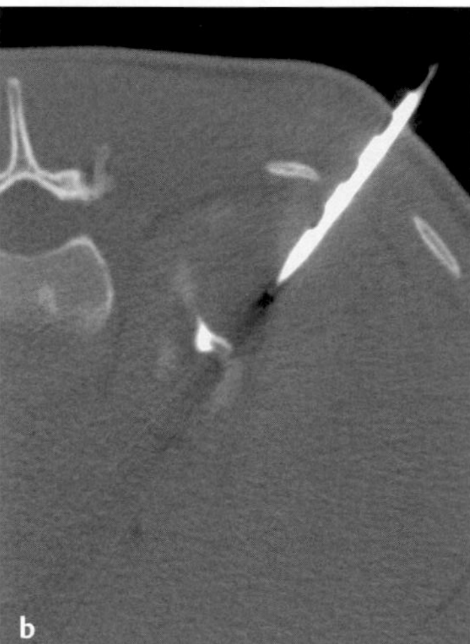

Fig. 1.22 a, b Drainage of a large abscess in the right kidney.

a Corticomedullary phase multislice CT obtained with the patient prone. Contrast enhancement of the abscess wall.

b CT-guided drainage of the abscess.

Clinical Aspects

- **Typical presentation**
  Flank pain (dull) • Raised temperature (low-grade fever to septicemic levels) • Pyuria • Raised levels of inflammatory markers.
- **Treatment options**
  - *Small intrarenal abscess:* May respond to high-dose antibiotics.
  - *Large and perinephric abscesses:* Large-caliber percutaneous drainage • Some patients may require open incision and drainage with antibiotic prophylaxis.
- **Course and prognosis**
  Complications: Perinephric abscess resulting from rupture into the Gerota fascia • Pyonephrosis in case of involvement of the renal pelvis • Retroperitoneal abscess if there is extension beyond the Gerota fascia • Hydronephrosis in case of obstruction • Chronic abscess.
- **What does the clinician want to know?**
  Diagnosis • Location • Presence of complications.

Differential Diagnosis

Cystic RCC	– Different signs and symptoms
Infected renal cyst	– Is associated with more severe inflammation of the surrounding parenchyma when complicated by renal abscess

Tips and Pitfalls

Renal abscess may be mistaken for RCC.

Selected References

Browne RF et al. Imaging of urinary tract infection in the adult. Eur Radiol 2004; 14 (Suppl 3): E168–183

Paterson A. Urinary tract infection: An update on imaging strategies. Eur Radiol 2004; 14 (Suppl 4): L89–100

Definition

- **Epidemiology**
  Most common manifestation of tuberculosis outside the lungs • Unilateral renal tuberculosis in 70% of cases.
- **Etiology**
  Pathogen: Mycobacterium tuberculosis • Hematogenous dissemination during acute primary pulmonary tuberculosis • Lymphohematogenous spread from an inactive primary lesion.
  Stages:
  - Initial parenchymal stage: Cortical renal lesion resembling early pulmonary infiltrate • May be followed by granuloma formation with scarring • Further course depends on the virulence of the organism, host immunity, and underlying renal conditions.
  - Ulcerocavernous stage: Extension to pelvicaliceal system • Ulceration and cavitation with papillary destruction • Communication with the collecting system and descending canalicular spread.
  - End stage: Progressive parenchymal loss • Tuberculous pyonephrosis or autonephrectomy (putty kidney).

Imaging Signs

- **Modality of choice**
  CT.
- **CT findings**
  Unenhanced CT: Calcifications • Scars.
  After intravenous contrast administration: In the initial stage, miliary tubercles may be visualized as rounded low-attenuating lesions • Kidney may be enlarged • Hydrocalices, ureteral strictures/dilatation, or pyonephrosis in more advanced disease • Putty kidney and shrinkage.
- **Intravenous pyelogram findings**
  Papillary destruction • Cavitation • Ureteral strictures/dilatations • Tuberculomas or residual scars (variable degree of calcification).

Clinical Aspects

- **Typical presentation**
  Low-grade fever • Symptoms of UTI (dysuria, hematuria, pyuria, flank pain) • History of pulmonary tuberculosis • Pathogen detection by PCR, cell culture, and tuberculin test.
- **Treatment options**
  Medical therapy: Antituberculous agents • *Surgical therapy:* Removal of scar tissue and repair of strictures.

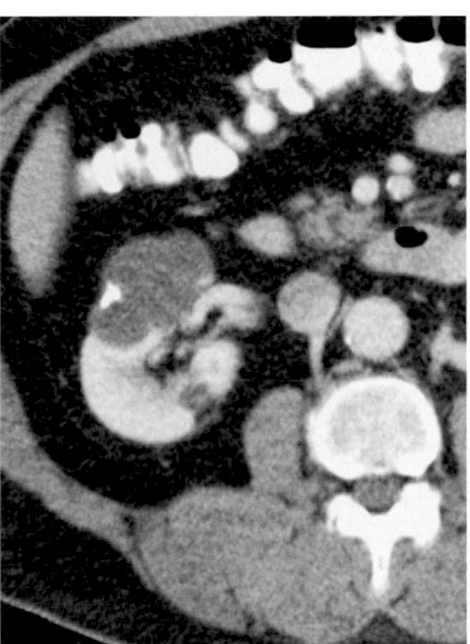

Fig. 1.23 Residuum of renal tuberculosis. Axial CT scan. Parenchymal thinning and eggshell calcification.

- **Course and prognosis**
  Complications: Descending infection, autonephrectomy, ureteral strictures.
- **What does the clinician want to know?**
  Confirmation of the tentative diagnosis • Morphologic extent.

Differential Diagnosis

Abacterial interstitial nephritis and other forms of UTI	– Pathogen isolation

Tips and Pitfalls

Although rare, renal tuberculosis must be considered in the differential diagnosis of conditions with similar radiologic changes.

Selected References

Murata Y et al. Abdominal macronodular tuberculomas: MR findings. J Comput Assist Tomogr 1996; 20: 643–646

Wang LJ et al. CT features of genitourinary tuberculosis. J Comput Assist Tomogr 1997; 21: 254–258

Definition

Nonneoplastic benign saclike structures containing fluid • Most commonly found in the renal cortex, less commonly in parenchymal or parapelvic location • Typically range in size from 2 cm to 5 cm (but may be as small as a few millimeters).

- **Epidemiology**
  Most common renal tumor • Frequency rises with age (> 50% of people older than 50 years) • Single or multiple • Unilateral or bilateral.
- **Etiology**
  Most renal cysts are of unknown origin • Association with von Hippel–Lindau disease and tuberous sclerosis.

Imaging Signs

- **Modality of choice**
  Ultrasound.
- **Pathognomonic findings**
  Spherical or slightly ovoid shape, homogeneous internal structure, and smooth margin.
- **Ultrasound findings**
  Absence of internal echoes • Posterior acoustic enhancement • No visible cyst wall.
- **CT findings**
  Unenhanced CT: Fluid attenuation • Smoothly demarcated lesion • No visible cyst wall.
  After intravenous contrast administration: Fluid attenuation (< 10 HU) • No enhancement.
- **MRI findings**
  - T1-weighted image: Homogeneous internal structure isointense to fluid • Low signal intensity.
  - T2-weighted image: Homogeneous internal structure isointense to fluid • High signal intensity.
  - T1-weighted image after contrast administration: No enhancement.
- **Intravenous pyelogram findings**
  Splaying of calices by smooth tumor.

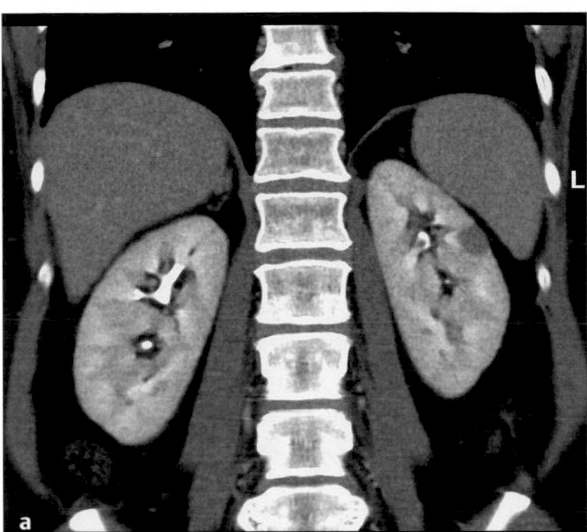

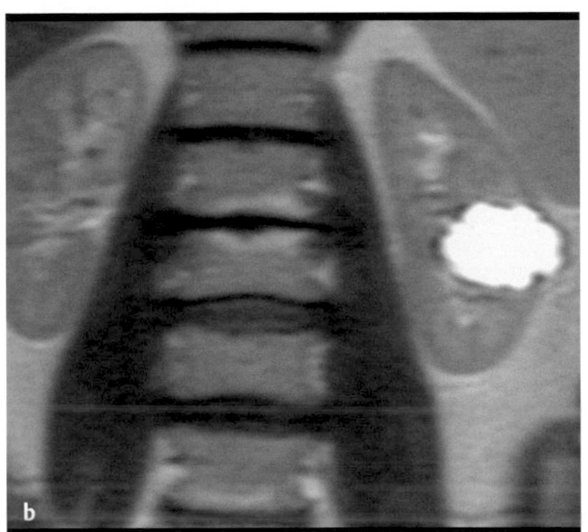

Fig. 1.24 a, b
Simple renal cysts.

a Simple cyst in the middle third of the left kidney. Coronal MPR from cortico-medullary phase multislice CT data. Homogeneous internal structure.

b Uncomplicated cyst. Unenhanced coronal T2-weighted MR image showing a slightly lobulated lesion.

Clinical Aspects

- **Typical presentation**
  Uncomplicated cysts are asymptomatic • Large or multiple parapelvic cysts can distort the pelvicaliceal system (rarely associated with segmental urinary obstruction) • An occasional large cyst may cause flank pain and can be palpated as a mass.
- **Treatment options**
  No treatment necessary in most cases • Large symptomatic cysts (rare) can be excised or treated by laparoscopic fenestration.
- **What does the clinician want to know?**
  Exclusion of complicated cyst • Exclusion of malignancy.

Differential Diagnosis

Complicated cysts	– Features such as intracystic hemorrhage or infection
Atypical cysts	– Calcification – Septa – Attenuation value > 20 HU
Renal abscess	– Higher attenuation than fluid – Wall thickness – Wall enhancement – Clinical presentation
Cystic RCC	– Septa – Wall thickness – Contrast enhancement

Tips and Pitfalls

Parapelvic cysts may be misinterpreted as urinary obstruction on ultrasound.

Selected References

Hartman DS et al. From the RSNA refresher courses: A practical approach to the cystic renal mass. Radiographics 2004; 24 (Suppl 1): S101–115

Israel GM, Bosniak MA. MR imaging of cystic renal masses. Magn Reson Imaging Clin North Am 2004; 12: 403–412

Definition

Cysts that do not meet the morphologic criteria of a simple, uncomplicated cyst.
Atypical cyst: Intracystic calcification and thickened wall • Higher viscosity of cyst fluid • Septa • Homogeneous internal structure and smooth wall.
Complicated cyst: Hemorrhagic cyst—simple cyst secondarily affected by hemorrhage due to trauma or hemorrhagic diathesis • Infected cyst—vesicoureteral reflux, hematogenous infection • Ruptured cyst.

Imaging Signs

- **Modality of choice**
  Ultrasound • CT • MRI.
- **Ultrasound findings**
  Higher echogenicity of cyst content • Septa • Thickened wall.
- **CT findings**
  Unenhanced CT:
  - *Complicated/atypical:* Attenuation of cyst fluid > 20 HU.
  - *Acute hemorrhage:* High attenuation.
  - *Chronic hemorrhage:* Heterogeneous appearance • Sediment may be present • Possible wall calcification.
  - *Infection:* Thickened wall • Higher attenuation of cyst fluid • Heterogeneous appearance • Gas inclusions • Septa may be present • Calcification in chronic infection.

  After intravenous contrast administration:
  - *Acute hemorrhage:* Low attenuation of cyst fluid in the cortical phase • High attenuation of fluid in the corticomedullary phase • Urographic phase—fluid level in the cyst if there is communication with the collecting system.
  - *Infection*: Enhancement of the thickened wall • Enhancement of cyst content • Fluid level • Gas inclusions.
  - *Ruptured cyst:* Heterogeneous appearance • Contrast uptake by perirenal hematoma.
- **MRI findings**
  - *Atypical:* T1-weighted image: slightly increased signal intensity of cyst fluid due to higher protein content • T2-weighted image: very high signal intensity • Homogeneous internal structure • Mural calcifications are seen as signal voids on T1- and T2-weighted images • T1-weighted image after intravenous contrast administration: no enhancement of the wall or fluid.
  - *Hemorrhage:* T1-weighted image: hyperintense or isointense, depending on age of hemorrhage and relaxation times of blood degradation products (methemoglobin) • T2-weighted image: hypointense, isointense, or hyperintense • T1-weighted image after intravenous contrast administration: no enhancement of the wall or contents.

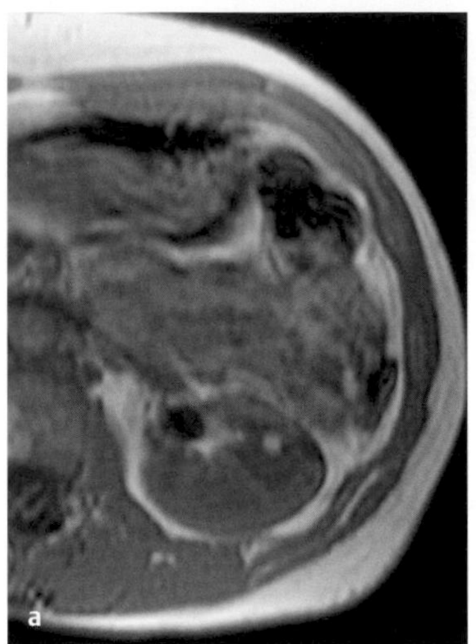

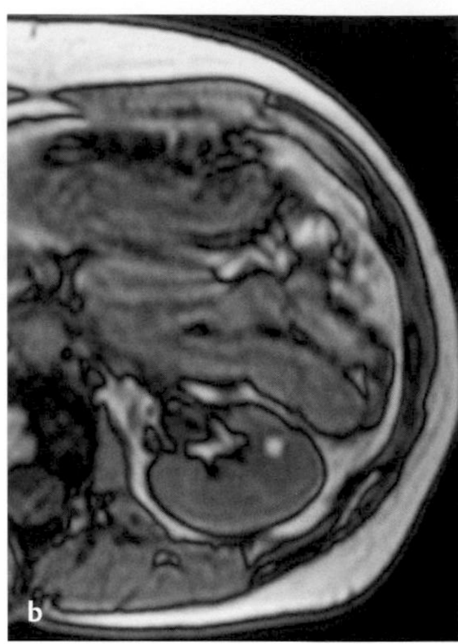

Fig. 1.25 a, b Small hemorrhagic cyst in the left kidney.
a T1-weighted in-phase GRE MR image. Lesion with high signal intensity.
b T1-weighted opposed-phase GRE image. No signal decrease at the interface between the lesion and surrounding normal renal parenchyma. Differential diagnosis: angiomyolipoma.

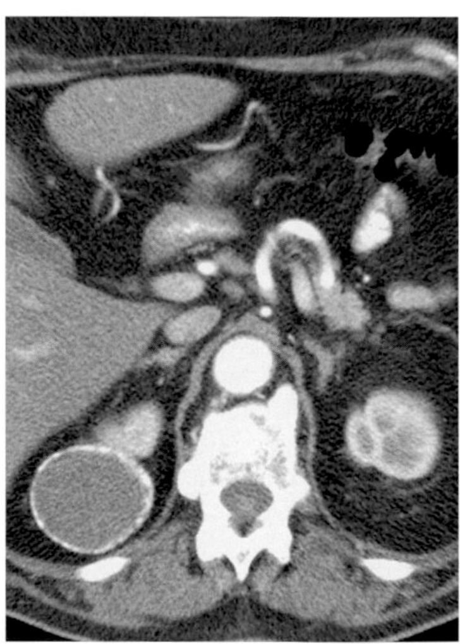

Fig. 1.26 Renal cyst with eggshell calcification. Axial multislice CT scan.

- *Infection:* T1-weighted image: higher signal of cyst fluid compared with uncomplicated cyst • T1-weighted image after intravenous contrast administration: heterogeneous enhancement.
- *Rupture:* Cyst appears heterogeneous • Perirenal hematoma.

Clinical Aspects

- **Typical presentation**
  Infected cyst: Fever, hematuria, urosepsis, flank pain.
- **Treatment options**
  Symptomatic treatment.
- **Course and prognosis**
  Follow-up of hemorrhagic or atypical cyst if there are no signs of infection or malignancy • *Ruptured or infected cyst:* Prognosis depends on complications.
- **What does the clinician want to know?**
  Diagnosis • Size • Exclusion of malignancy.

Differential Diagnosis

Renal abscess	– Wall enhancement – Reactive inflammation of surrounding parenchyma
Echinococcal cyst	– Calcifications – Septa – Wall enhancement – Other manifestations
Polycystic kidney disease	– Bilateral – Parenchymal displacement
Cystadenoma	– Visualization of capsule (30%) – No solid tumor components
Cystic RCC	– Irregular contour – Solid, typically nodular, tumor components

Tips and Pitfalls

Malignancy must be excluded, if necessary using different imaging modalities.

Selected References

Hartman DS et al. From the RSNA refresher courses: A practical approach to the cystic renal mass. Radiographics 2004; 24 (Suppl 1): S101–115

Israel GM, Bosniak MA. MR imaging of cystic renal masses. Magn Reson Imaging Clin North Am 2004; 12: 403–412

Definition

A condition characterized by multiple renal cysts with marked/massive enlargement of the kidneys.

- **Epidemiology**
  - *Autosomal dominant polycystic kidney disease* (ADPKD): Adult form • Common • Incidence of 1:400 to 1:1000
  - *Autosomal recessive polycystic kidney disease* (ARPKD): Infantile form • Rare • Incidence of 1:10000 to 1:40000
- **Etiology**
  Multisystemic condition characterized by cystic destruction of the renal parenchyma and progressive renal failure.
  ADPKD: Polycystic kidneys.
  Extrarenal manifestations:
  - Cysts: Hepatic cysts (100%), pancreatic cysts (10%), arachnoid cysts; associated cysts in the bladder, ovaries, or testicles are rare.
  - Diverticulosis/diverticulitis of the colon.
  - Intracranial aneurysms (40%), coronary artery and aortic aneurysms.
  - Cardiac valve defects.

  ARPKD: Renal manifestation: Cysts typically measure only a few millimeters • Extrarenal manifestations: Congenital liver fibrosis, hepatosplenomegaly.

Imaging Signs

- **Modality of choice**
  MRI.
- **General**
  Multiple cysts • Enlarged kidneys • Enlargement may be asymmetric.
- **MRI findings**
  - *Simple cysts:* T1-weighted image: low signal intensity/fluid isointensity of cyst contents • T2-weighted image: high signal intensity/fluid isointensity of cyst contents • T1-weighted image after intravenous contrast administration: no enhancement.
  - *Intracystic hemorrhage:* T1-weighted image: typically high signal intensity due to presence of blood degradation products (methemoglobin) • T2-weighted image: variable intensity.
  - *Infected cysts:* T1-weighted image after intravenous contrast administration: wall enhancement • Gas inclusions.
  - *Rupture:* T1-weighted image after intravenous contrast administration: wall enhancement • Perirenal hematoma.
- **CT findings**
  - *Simple cysts:* Homogeneous with fluid attenuation on unenhanced scans • No enhancement after contrast administration.

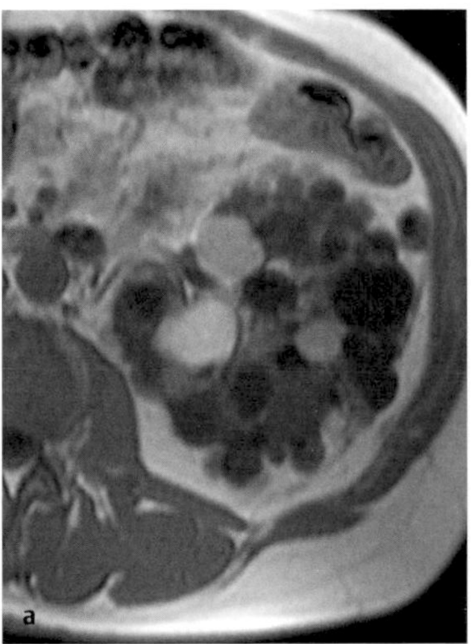

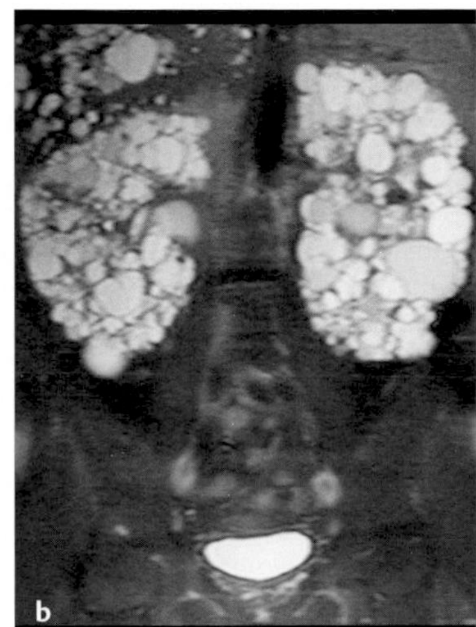

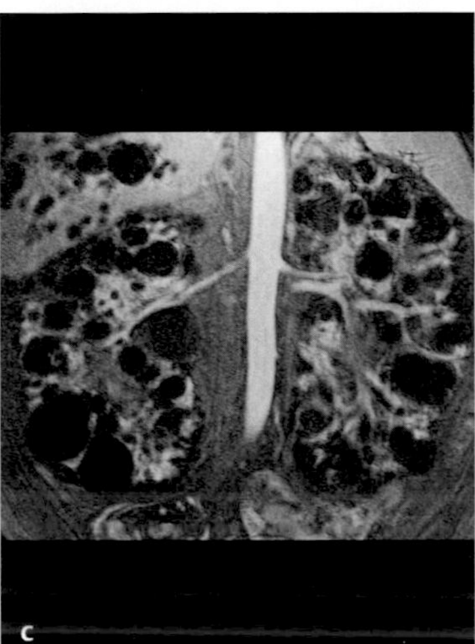

Fig. 1.27 a–c Bilateral polycystic kidney disease with hemorrhage into some cysts.

- **a** Axial T1-weighted MR image.
- **b** Fat-saturated T2-weighted MR image.
- **c** Fat-saturated T1-weighted MR image after intravenous contrast administration.

- *Intracystic hemorrhage:* Fresh blood has high attenuation on unenhanced scans • Becomes hypodense relative to adjacent parenchyma after contrast administration.
- *Infected cysts and rupture:* As on MRI.

Clinical Aspects

- **Typical presentation, course and prognosis**
  ADPKD: Onset typically between 20 and 50 years • Symptoms vary with severity of renal changes and complications • Flank pain if there is obstruction or calculus • Hematuria • Rupture of cyst/hemorrhage into cyst • Hypertension • Recurrent UTI • Urolithiasis • Progressive renal failure • Symptoms associated with extrarenal manifestations.
  ARPKD: Symptoms depend on progression of renal failure and severity of hepatic involvement; high mortality in childhood • Arterial hypertension • Portal hypertension • Complications such as gastrointestinal bleeding.
- **Treatment options**
  Symptomatic treatment, e.g., of hypertension or UTI • Kidney transplant.
- **What does the clinician want to know?**
  Size of the kidneys • Displacement • Presence of complicated cysts.

Differential Diagnosis

Acquired cystic kidney disease	– Complication of chronic renal failure and hemodialysis – Secondary cyst formation in atrophic kidneys – At least four cysts must be present to diagnose acquired cystic kidney disease – Rare complications—hematuria, development of RCC
Nephronophthisis–medullary cystic kidney disease complex	– Congenital disorder characterized by cyst formation at the corticomedullary junction and interstitial fibrosis – Absence of calcifications, demonstrated histologically and possibly by imaging, distinguishes this condition from medullary sponge kidney – Clinical presentation—progressive renal failure in childhood

Tips and Pitfalls

Acquired cystic kidney disease must not be mistaken for polycystic kidney disease.

Selected References

Lonergan GJ et al. Autosomal recessive polycystic kidney disease: radiologic-pathologic correlation. Radiographics 2000; 20: 837–855

Mosetti MA et al. Autosomal dominant polycystic kidney disease: MR imaging evaluation using current techniques. J Magn Reson Imaging 2003; 18: 210–215

Definition

A benign mesenchymal tumor of the kidney composed of varying amounts of mature adipose tissue, smooth muscle, and blood vessels.

- **Epidemiology**
  Relatively common tumor with a prevalence of 0.3–3%. More common in women.
- **Etiology**
  Hamartoma a few centimeters in size • Typically unilateral • May in rare cases invade the renal vein • Bilateral angiomyolipoma in patients with tuberous sclerosis.

Imaging Signs

- **Modality of choice**
  Ultrasound • MRI.
- **Pathognomonic findings**
  Well-defined, fatty mass in the kidney • One or more lesions • Fatty component in the center or periphery • No calcification.
- **Ultrasound findings**
  Highly echogenic mass • Smoothly demarcated.
- **MRI findings**
  T1-weighted/T2-weighted images: typically high signal intensity specific for fat • Fat-saturated T2-weighted or double-echo T1-weighted (opposed-phase) sequence: signal decrease • Contrast-enhanced images provide no additional information for the differential diagnosis.
- **CT findings**
  Intrarenal areas of fat attenuation on unenhanced scans point to the diagnosis • Cortical phase after intravenous contrast administration: enhancement varies with tumor size and vascularity.

Clinical Aspects

- **Typical presentation**
  Usually asymptomatic and detected incidentally • Patients with large angiomyolipomas may have symptoms because of bleeding.
- **Treatment options**
  Surgical resection or embolization of symptomatic tumors.
- **Course and prognosis**
  Follow-up.
- **What does the clinician want to know?**
  Diagnosis • Exclusion of malignancy.

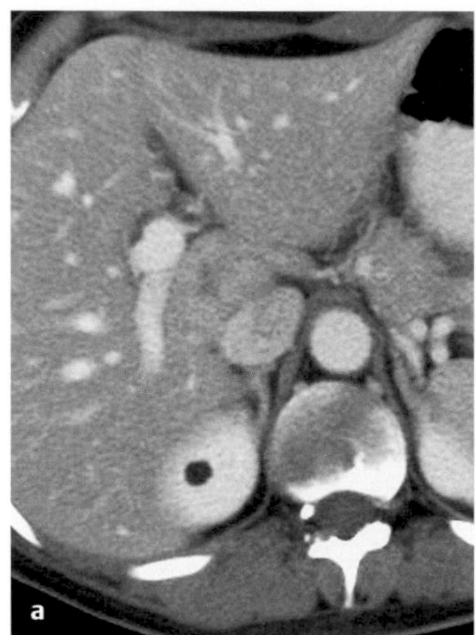

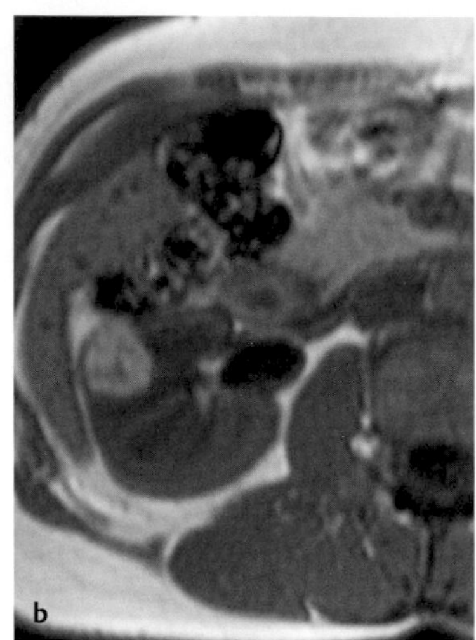

Fig. 1.28 a–c Angiomyolipoma of the right kidney.

a Axial multislice CT. Corticomedullary phase scan showing a small hypodense mass at the upper pole of the right kidney.

b Unenhanced MRI, axial T1-weighted GRE sequence. In-phase image showing a hyperintense mass.

c MRI, axial T1-weighted GRE sequence. Opposed-phase image showing a hypointense interface between the renal parenchyma and fatty angiomyolipoma.

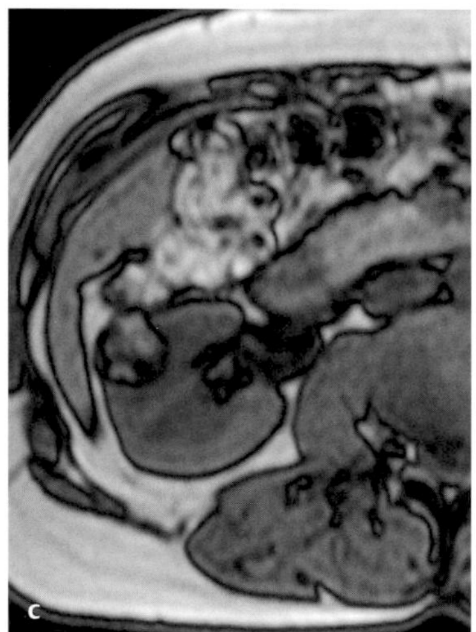

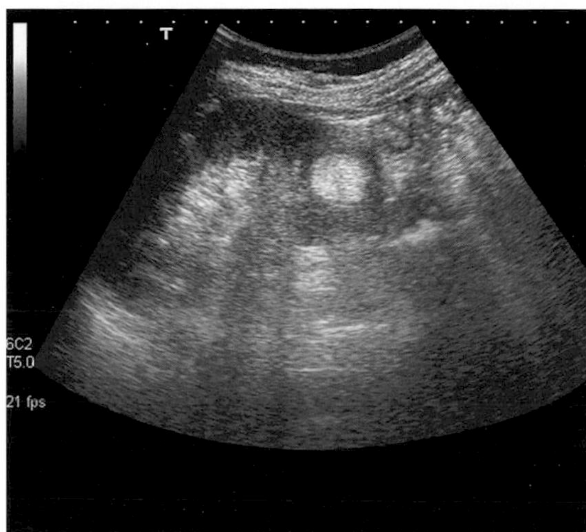

Fig. 1.29 Angiomyolipoma. Ultrasound. Highly echogenic mass with smooth margins.

Differential Diagnosis

Hemorrhagic cyst	- Moderately high signal on T1-weighted/ T2-weighted images - No hypointense interface between the lesion and surrounding parenchyma on opposed-phase GRE images
RCC or metastasis from RCC with fatty components	- Very rare - Can be differentiated on the basis of its contrast enhancement pattern

Tips and Pitfalls

Carefully look for the fatty components, which are the hallmark of angiomyolipoma.

Selected References

Kim JK et al. Angiomyolipoma with minimal fat: differentiation from renal cell carcinoma at biphasic helical CT. Radiology 2004; 230: 677–684

Strunk HM. Renal angiomyolipoma. Ultraschall Med 2002; 23: 367–372

Definition

A well-differentiated tubulopapillary renal cell carcinoma.

- **Etiology**
  Arises from the proximal tubular epithelium.

Imaging Signs

- **Modality of choice**
  CT • MRI.
- **General**
  Most hypovascular RCCs are detected incidentally • Usually subcapsular • Smoothly marginated • Typically homogeneous.
- **MRI findings**
  T1- and T2-weighted images: isointense/hypointense • T1-weighted image after intravenous contrast administration: tumor hypointense to parenchyma.
- **CT findings**
  CT after intravenous contrast administration: hypodense to parenchyma in the corticomedullary phase.

Clinical Aspects

- **Typical presentation**
  Usually asymptomatic.
- **Treatment options**
  Surgical resection • Radiofrequency ablation.
- **What does the clinician want to know?**
  Diagnosis • Extent • Signs of malignancy.

Differential Diagnosis

Oncocytoma	– Differentiation may be difficult if spoke-wheel enhancement is absent

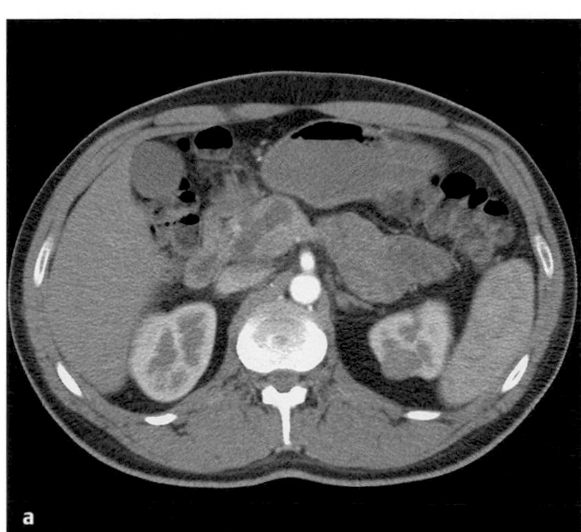

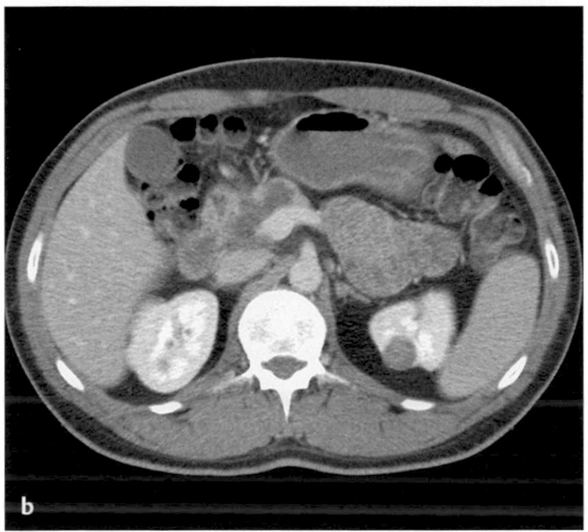

Fig. 1.30 a, b Highly differentiated hypovascular RCC in the upper third of the left kidney.

a Contrast-enhanced axial multislice CT during the cortical phase.

b Corticomedullary phase.

Definition

A usually benign neoplasm that arises in the tubular epithelium and is composed of oncocytes; characterized by very slow growth and rare metastatic spread • *Synonym:* Proximal tubular adenoma with oncocytic features.

- **Epidemiology**
  Accounts for 5% of all renal tumors.
- **Etiology**
  Mutation of mitochondrial DNA.

Imaging Signs

- **Modality of choice**
  CT • MRI.
- **Pathognomonic findings**
  Usually detected incidentally • Characteristic central scar • Spoke-wheel configuration of vessels (up to 80% of renal oncocytomas) • Otherwise homogeneous internal structure • Well-demarcated mass.
- **CT findings**
  CT after intravenous contrast administration: hypervascular tumor (cortical phase) • Spoke-wheel pattern • Central scar.
- **MRI findings**
  T1-weighted image: hypointense/isointense • T2-weighted image: hyperintense • T1-weighted image after intravenous contrast administration: hypervascular tumor in the arterial phase, spoke-wheel pattern.
- **Angiographic findings**
  Spoke-wheel pattern (up to 80%).

Clinical Aspects

- **Typical presentation**
  Asymptomatic.
- **Treatment options**
  Surgical resection should be considered because oncocytomas can occasionally metastasize and their radiologic features do not allow reliable differentiation from RCC.
- **Course and prognosis**
  Good after surgical resection.
- **What does the clinician want to know?**
  Diagnosis • Extent.

Differential Diagnosis

Well-differentiated RCC	– Often impossible to distinguish from oncocytoma

Selected References

Harmon WJ et al. Renal oncocytoma: magnetic resonance imaging characteristics. J Urol 1996; 155: 863–867

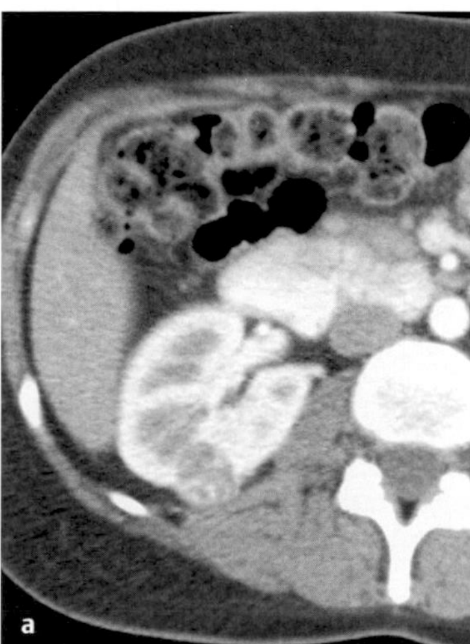

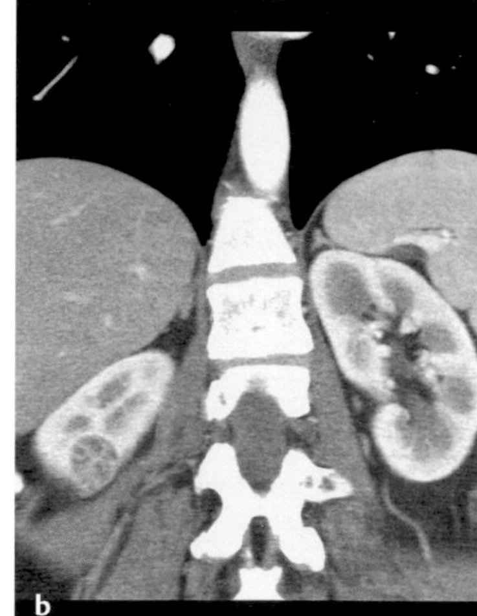

Fig. 1.31 a, b Oncocytoma in the posterior aspect of the middle third of the right kidney. Spoke-wheel-like enhancement in the cortical phase.
a Axial scan in the cortical phase obtained with biphasic multislice CT.
b Coronal MPR of the cortical phase.

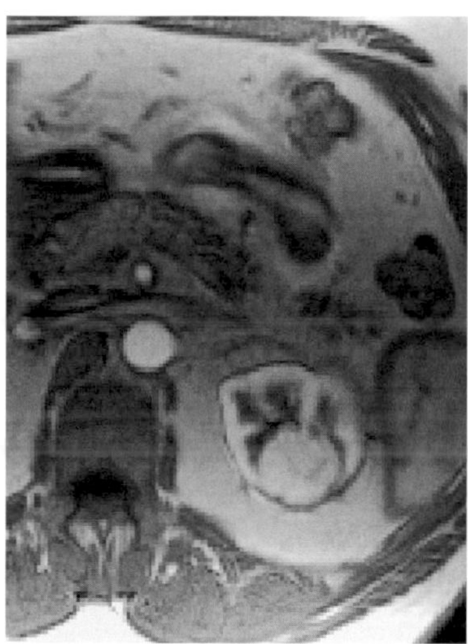

Fig. 1.32 Oncocytoma in the upper third of the left kidney. Axial T1-weighted GRE MR image obtained during the cortical phase after intravenous contrast administration.

Definition

A malignant epithelial tumor of the renal parenchyma usually arising in the renal poles • The cut surface shows a yellowish tumor due to fatty components, which are interspersed with hemorrhagic and necrotic areas • *Synonym:* Renal adenocarcinoma.

► **Epidemiology**

Accounts for over 85% of all solid renal tumors and 3% of all malignancies • Most RCCs present in the sixth decade of life.

Histologic subtypes:

- *Clear cell* (80%): Proximal tubular cells.
- *Chromophilic* (10%): Proximal tubular cells • Papillary growth pattern.
- *Chromophobe* (5%): Intercalated cells of the collecting ducts.
- *Spindle cell* (1%): Sarcomatoid • Poor prognosis.
- *Collecting duct* (Bellini duct): Poor prognosis.

Association with von Hippel–Lindau disease and tuberous sclerosis.

Imaging Signs

► **Modality of choice**

Biphasic CT/MRI after intravenous contrast administration • Ultrasound.

► **Pathognomonic findings**

Solid tumor of the renal cortex with rich vascular supply • Imaging appearance of large RCCs varies according to the relative amounts of necrotic, cystic, and fatty elements • Pseudocapsule.

► **CT findings**

Unenhanced CT: Isodense • Tumor may produce bulging of the renal contour • Areas of decreased and increased attenuation due to hemorrhage and necrosis • Calcification is rare.

After intravenous contrast administration: Biphasic scan in patients with suspected RCC, otherwise monophasic scan with acquisition of the corticomedullary phase • Typically hypervascularized • Most RCCs enhance significantly in the cortical phase • Hypodense in the corticomedullary phase • Large tumors appear inhomogeneous (necrosis, hemorrhage) • Invasion of the renal sinus or renal vein • In case of vascular invasion, a tumor/appositional thrombus extending up into the right atrium may be seen (more common in RCC of the right kidney).

► **MRI findings**

- T1- and T2-weighted images: Signal intensity varies with histology, typically hypointense to isointense • Inhomogeneous structure • Pseudocapsule.
- T1-weighted image after intravenous contrast administration: Marked but inhomogeneous enhancement • Chromophilic RCCs show less enhancement.

► **Ultrasound findings**

Heterogeneous mass • Typically isoechoic, but also hypoechoic or hyperechoic • Color Doppler ultrasound: highly vascular lesion and high flow velocity.

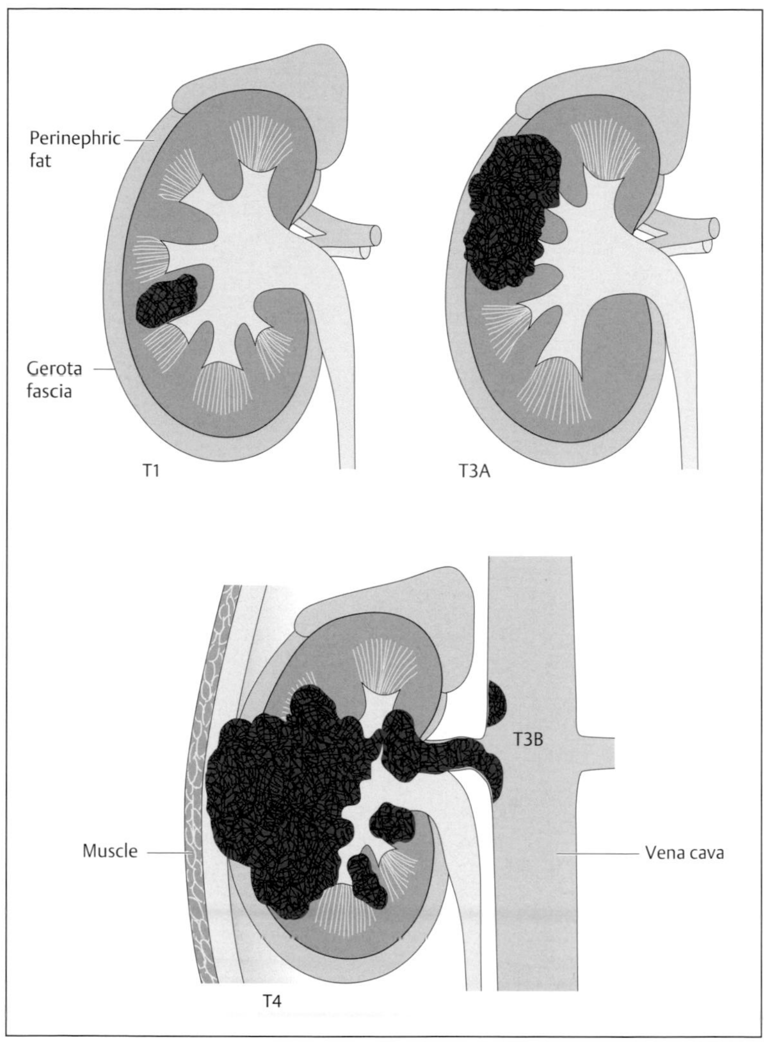

Fig. 1.33 Staging of renal cell carcinoma.

T1 Small tumor (≤ 7 cm) confined to the kidney

T2 Large tumor (> 7 cm) confined to the kidney

T3A Tumor invades perinephric fat/adrenal gland

T3B Tumor extends into the renal vein/inferior vena cava

T4 Tumor invades adjacent organs (other than adrenal)

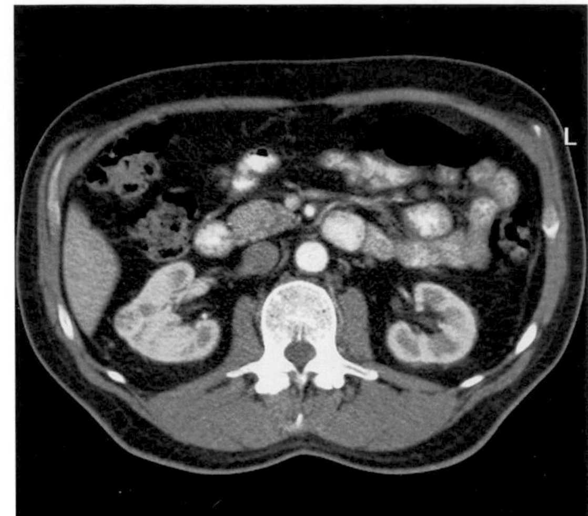

Fig. 1.34 Small renal cell carcinoma in the middle third of the right kidney. There is no involvement of the renal sinus. Multislice CT scan in the cortical phase.

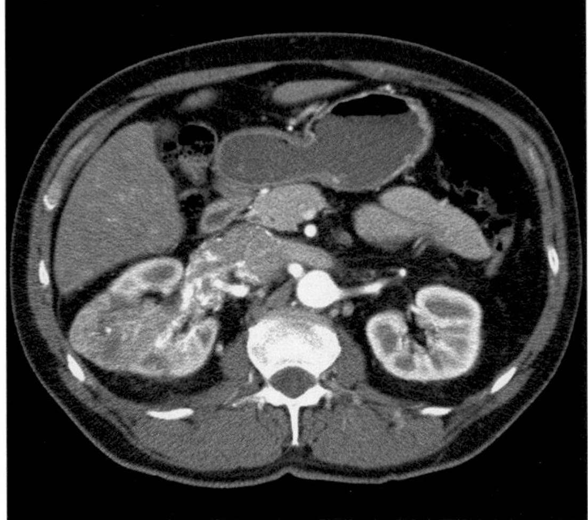

Fig. 1.35 Large renal cell carcinoma extending into the renal vein and large tumor thrombus in the inferior vena cava. Axial multislice CT scan.

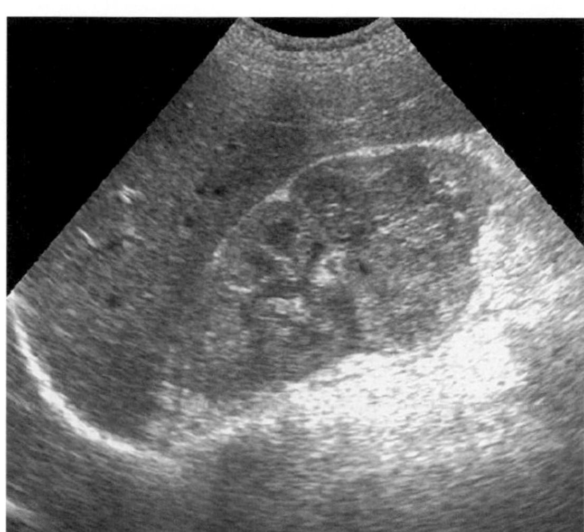

Fig. 1.36 Renal cell carcinoma. B-mode ultrasound scan.

- **Intravenous pyelogram findings**
  Bulging of the renal outline • Distortion of the pelvicaliceal system.
- **CTA and MRA**
  To evaluate the vascular status in patients scheduled for endoscopic nephrectomy.

Clinical Aspects

- **Typical presentation**
  Many RCCs remain asymptomatic until they are advanced • Hematuria • Flank pain • Weight loss • *Paraneoplastic syndrome:* Arterial hypertension (renin), polycythemia (EPO), hypercalcemia (PTH), Cushing syndrome (ACTH) • *Metastases:* Lymphatic spread; hematogenous spread (via the vena cava) to the lungs, bones, liver, brain, contralateral kidney, adrenals, and pancreas • Metastases from RCC are often detected before the primary is diagnosed.
- **Treatment options**
  Nephrectomy/partial nephrectomy (both can be performed laparoscopically) • Oncologic treatment (immunotherapy).
- **Course and prognosis**
  Five-year survival rates by tumor stage:
  - Tumor confined to the kidney (T1/T2, N0, M0): 70–80%.
  - Local tumor extension beyond the kidney (T3, N0–N2, M0): 20–60%.
  - Distant metastases (all T and N stages, M1): < 10%.
- **What does the clinician want to know?**
  Diagnosis • Accurate staging • Presence of tumor thrombus.

Differential Diagnosis

Angiomyolipoma	– If unenhanced CT demonstrates fatty components, contrast administration or MRI will provide further clarification
Adenoma/oncocytoma	– Cannot be distinguished from well-differentiated RCC
Hemorrhagic renal cyst	– Biphasic MRI or CT
Renal abscess	– Clinical signs and symptoms, urinalysis
Lymphoma	– Localized lymphoma is difficult to distinguish from well-differentiated RCC

Tips and Pitfalls

Parenchymal isthmus may be misinterpreted on ultrasound • Small RCCs may be overlooked on cortical phase cross-sectional images.

Selected References

Helenon O et al. Ultrasound of renal tumors. Eur Radiol 2001; 11: 1890–1901
Sheth S et al. Current concepts in the diagnosis and management of renal cell carcinoma: role of multidetector CT and three-dimensional CT. Radiographics 2001; 21: S237–254

Definition

Cystadenoma: Cystic mass of the kidney without radiologic signs of malignancy • Consists of multiple noncommunicating cysts, which may contain septa • Capsule in 30% of cases • Rare tumor of unclear etiology (hamartoma, dysplasia) • *Synonyms:* Multilocular renal cyst and benign cystic nephroma.
Cystic RCC: Cystic renal mass with signs of malignancy.

Imaging Signs

- **Modality of choice**
  Ultrasound • CT • MRI.
- **Ultrasound findings**
  Renal mass consisting of multiple anechoic cysts • Possible capsule • Solid components may be seen in cystic RCC.
- **CT and MRI findings**
  CT and T1-weighted MRI after intravenous contrast administration:
  - *Cystadenoma:* Capsule in 30% of cases • Multilocular tumor • Thick septa and capsule take up contrast • No enhancement of cyst fluid.
  - *Cystic RCC:* Solid nodular wall components • Wall enhancement • Thick septa • Ill-defined margin.

Clinical Aspects

- **Typical presentation**
  Symptoms are usually nonspecific • Flank pain • Hematuria.
- **Treatment options**
  - *Cystadenoma:* Tumor resection if this can be accomplished by partial nephrectomy.
  - *Cystic RCC:* Resection • Oncologic treatment.
- **Course and prognosis**
  Depend on degree of malignancy of cystic RCC and response to treatment.
- **What does the clinician want to know?**
  Diagnosis • Extent • Malignancy.

Differential Diagnosis

Renal abscess	– Wall enhancement – Reactive inflammation of surrounding parenchyma

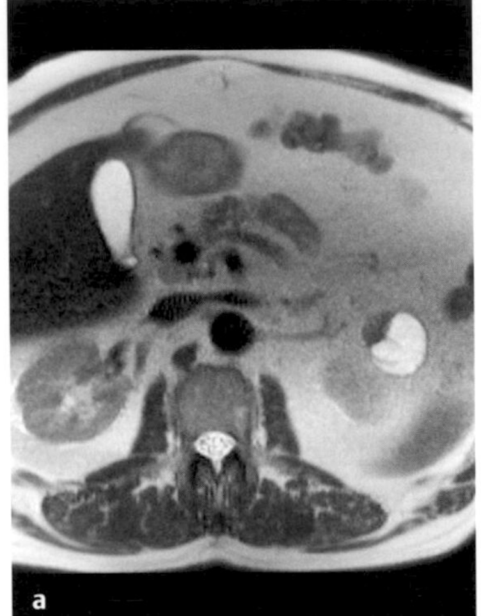

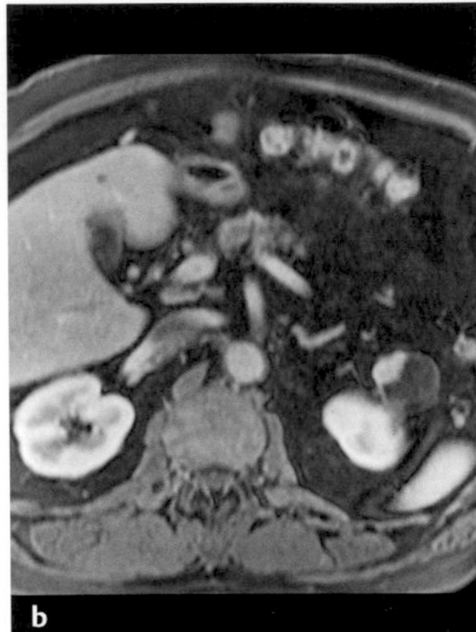

Fig. 1.37 a–c Cystic renal cell carcinoma in the upper third of the left kidney. Tumor in the renal cortex consisting of cystic and solid components.

- **a** Unenhanced T2-weighted MR image.
- **b** Cortical phase T1-weighted image after intravenous contrast medium.
- **c** Corticomedullary phase T1-weighted image after intravenous contrast medium.

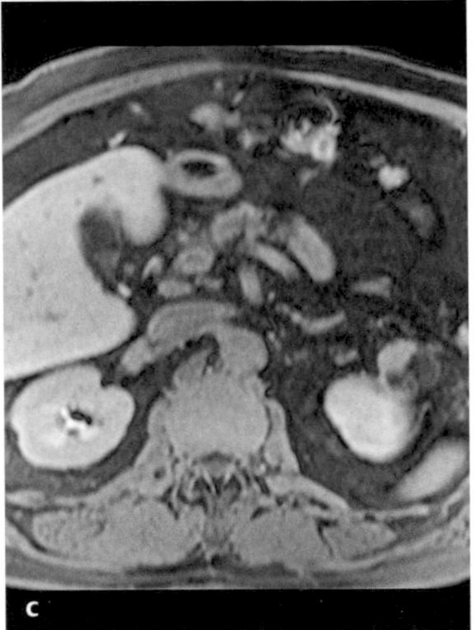

Tips and Pitfalls

Small solid tumor parts may be overlooked on ultrasound • Unclear cases are resolved by biphasic CT/MRI.

Selected References

Benjaminov O et al. Enhancing component on CT to predict malignancy in cystic renal masses and interobserver agreement of different CT features. AJR 2006; 186: 665–672

Israel GM, Bosniak MA. MR imaging of cystic renal masses. Magn Reson Imaging Clin N Am 2004; 12: 403–412

Definition

Renal lymphomas typically occur as a manifestation of systemic disease • Hematogenous dissemination of lymphoma to the kidney or contiguous extension from retroperitoneal disease.

- **Epidemiology**
  Primary renal lymphoma is very rare • Secondary renal involvement in 30–60% of patients with non-Hodgkin lymphoma.
- **Etiology**
  Hematogenous spread to the kidneys occurs late in the course of the disease • Renal involvement more common in patients with NHL, lymphoma of higher malignancy, diffuse lymphoma, and lymphoma development after organ transplantation > • Infiltrative interstitial growth sparing parenchymal structures.

Imaging Signs

- **Modality of choice**
  Biphasic CT/MRI after intravenous contrast administration • Ultrasound.
- **General**
  Typically multiple lymphomas in both kidneys • Lesions usually measure 1–3 cm • Diffuse involvement with enlargement of the kidney • Demonstration of a single well-defined lymphoma is rare • Invasion from outside/contiguous extension from the retroperitoneum.
- **CT findings**
  After intravenous contrast administration: Hypovascular lesions • Low attenuation relative to surrounding parenchyma • Irregular lesions • Diffuse lymphoma is indicated by diffusely reduced parenchymal enhancement and reduced excretion • Enlargement of the kidney or capsular bulging • Diffuse infiltration of perinephric tissue may be present • Involvement of the pelvicaliceal system can be assessed in the corticomedullary and urographic phases.
- **MRI findings**
  T1-weighted image: isointense or hypointense lesion • T2-weighted image: hypointense lesion • T1-weighted image after intravenous contrast administration: lower enhancement of lymphoma compared to parenchyma (see CT after intravenous contrast administration).
- **Ultrasound findings**
  Hypoechoic masses.

Clinical Aspects

- **Typical presentation**
  Nonspecific and related to the site of lymphoma (e.g., urinary obstruction) • Possible flank pain • Hematuria • Palpable tumor.
- **Treatment options**
  Chemotherapy • Resection is not an option in most cases because of advanced tumor stage at presentation.

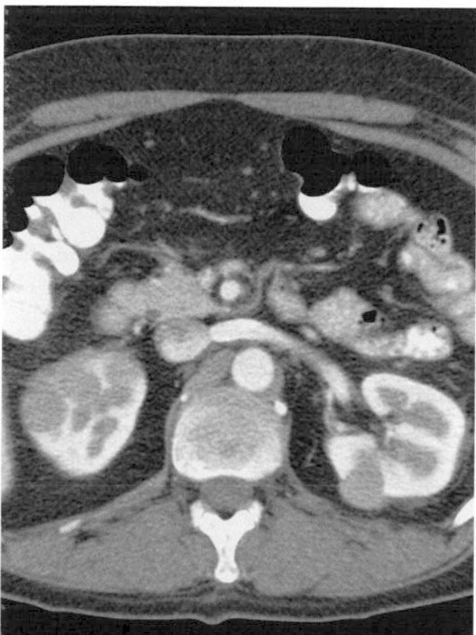

Fig. 1.38 Multiple lymphomas in both kidneys. Cortical phase axial multislice CT scan. Rounded lesions with lower attenuation than renal parenchyma.

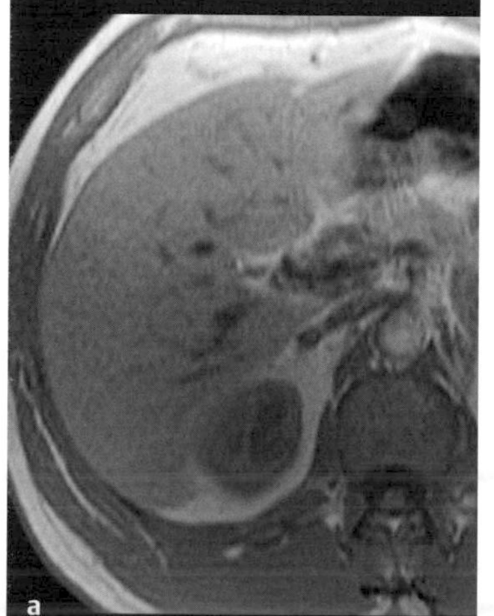

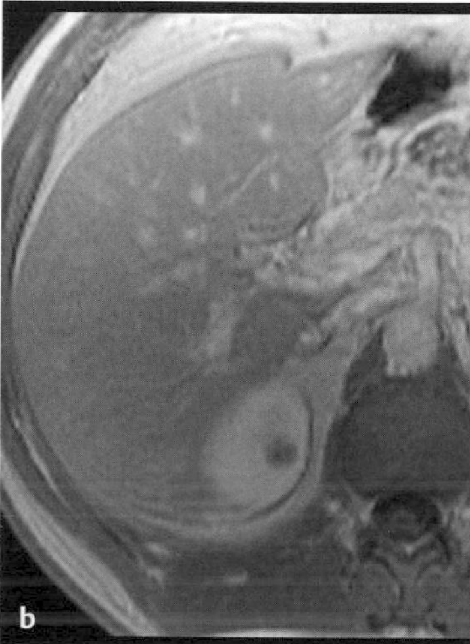

Fig. 1.39 a, b Lymphoma in the upper pole of the right kidney.

a Unenhanced axial T1-weighted MR image. Moderately hypointense lymphoma.

b T1-weighted MR image after intravenous contrast administration. The lesion becomes more conspicuous on the corticomedullary phase image.

- **Course and prognosis**
  Depend on extent of renal lymphoma and tumor stage.
- **What does the clinician want to know?**
  Diagnosis • Pattern of involvement • Perinephric extension • Complications.

Differential Diagnosis

RCC	– Most renal lymphomas are homogeneous and poorly defined. Focal lymphoma is difficult to differentiate from RCC

Tips and Pitfalls

Diffuse renal lymphoma may escape detection by CT or MRI even if a biphasic protocol is used.

Selected References

Sheeran SR, Sussman SK. Renal lymphoma: spectrum of CT findings and potential mimics. AJR 1998; 171: 1067–1072

Urban BA, Fishman EK. Renal lymphoma: CT patterns with emphasis on helical CT. Radiographics 2000; 20: 197–212

Definition

Phakomatoses are groups of diseases inherited as autosomal dominant traits and characterized by the development of hamartomas in various tissues • *Synonym:* Neurocutaneous syndromes.

- **Epidemiology**
  Neurofibromatosis type I: Also known as von Recklinghausen disease • Chromosome 17 q • Prevalence: 1:3000.
  Tuberous sclerosis: Also known as Bourneville–Pringle disease • Chromosome 9 q/16 q • *Prevalence:* 10:100 000.
  Von Hippel–Lindau disease: Chromosome 3 p • *Prevalence:* 0.6:100 000.
- **Etiology**
  Neurofibromatosis type I: Peripheral form • Café-au-lait spots • Neurofibromas • Iris hamartomas (Lisch nodules) • Optic glioma • Cerebellar astrocytomas • High incidence of Wilms tumor • Pheochromocytoma.
  Tuberous sclerosis: Adenoma sebaceum • Shagreen patches • Subungual fibromas (Koenen tumors) • Tubers (glial hamartomas) • Subependymal glial nodules • Cardiac rhabdomyoma • Pulmonary lymphangiomatosis • Seizures and mental retardation • Multitude of renal abnormalities • A patient with bilateral angiomyolipomas has an 80–90% likelihood of tuberous sclerosis • Rare association with RCC • Cystic kidneys.
  Von Hippel–Lindau disease: Hemangioblastomas of the retina and cerebellum, less commonly of the spinal cord • Pheochromocytoma • 40% of patients have renal angiomas • 30% have RCC (mostly clear cell subtype and often bilateral) • Renal cysts in 30% of patients, often associated with pancreatic cysts.

Imaging Signs

- **Modality of choice**
  Ultrasound • CT • MRI for precise characterization.
- **Findings**
  See also sections on angiomyolipoma, renal cysts, and renal cell carcinoma.
  Angiomyolipomas: Multiple, sometimes very large, hamartomas in both kidneys.
  RCC: Often bilateral.

Clinical Aspects

- **Treatment options**
  Symptomatic treatment • Tumor resection.
- **Course and prognosis**
  Depend on tumor stage in patients with RCC.
- **What does the clinician want to know?**
  Diagnosis • Tumor extent.

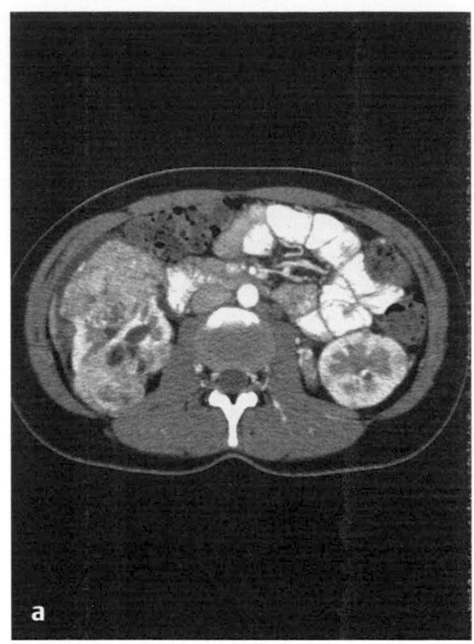

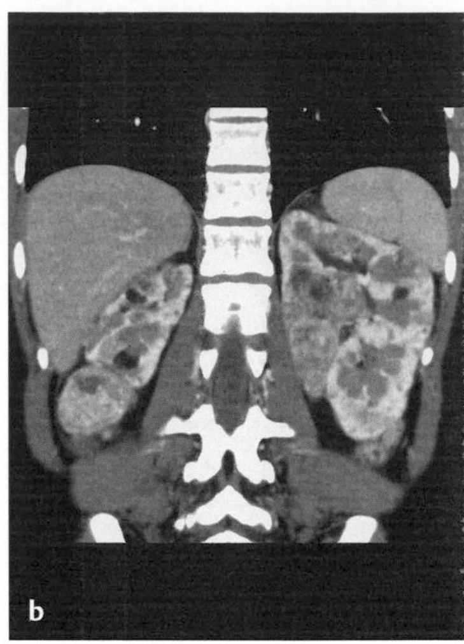

Fig. 1.40 a, b Multiple large angiomyolipomas in both kidneys in a patient with tuberous sclerosis.
a Cortical phase axial multislice CT scan after contrast administration.
b Coronal MPR from multislice CT data.

Differential Diagnosis

Renal cell carcinoma	– Bilateral RCC and neurologic symptoms suggest phakomatosis
Angiomyolipoma	– Multiple angiomyolipomas suggest phakomatosis, especially when bilateral

Selected References

Hes FJ, Feldberg MA. Von Hippel–Lindau disease: strategies in early detection (renal-, adrenal-, pancreatic masses). Eur Radiol 1999; 9: 598–610

Definition

- **Epidemiology**
  A kidney transplant is 50–60% less expensive than long-term hemodialysis over a 10-year period • Living donor kidneys constitute about 35% of all kidney transplants in the USA • Slight increase in kidney transplants in recent years.
- **Kidney donation and transplantation process**
  Prerequisites: Diagnosis of irreversible brain death and consent to organ donation by the deceased or their family • Consent also required for living donation • Eurotransplant (Leiden, the Netherlands) is the largest organ allocation network in Europe • Organ allocation criteria established in accordance with legal regulations • Criteria ensure optimal success and fair allocation • Medical checkup of living donors.
  Preparation: Blood group determination • Tissue typing—MHC and HLA antigens on chromosome 6, preformed antibodies.
  Preoperative radiologic workup: Chest and pelvic radiographs; abdominal ultrasound, Doppler ultrasound, ultrasound of the neck and iliac vessels • Biphasic MRA or CTA for evaluation of vascular anatomy in potential living donors and recipients.
  Absolute contraindications: Active malignancy • HIV infection and life expectancy of less than 2 years • Noncompliance • High probability of operative mortality.
  Relative contraindications: Malignant disease with tumor control • Active or chronic infection.
  Surgery: En bloc retrieval of donor kidney • Extraperitoneal implantation in the right or left iliac fossa • In general, end-to-side anastomosis to the external iliac artery/vein • Intravesical implantation of the transplant ureter, rarely extravesical implantation • Immunosuppression.

Imaging Signs

- **Modality of choice**
  Ultrasound.
- **Transplant follow-up (B-mode and color Doppler ultrasound)**
  Graft size • Resistance index • Pulsatility index • Evaluation of arterial and venous anastomoses.
- **CT and MRI findings**
  CT is indicated if there is acute bleeding • MR IVP is indicated to evaluate arterial kinking stenosis, to exclude urinary obstruction, and to detect urinoma.

Fig. 1.41 a, b
Second postoperative day after kidney transplant. Color Doppler ultrasound. Adequate arterial perfusion throughout the kidney graft. Normal resistance index.

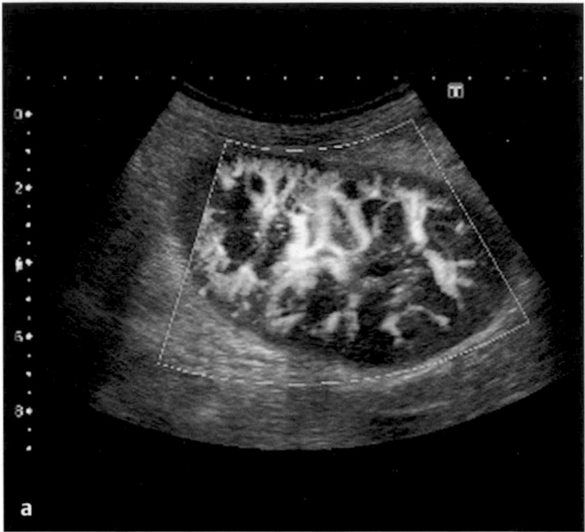

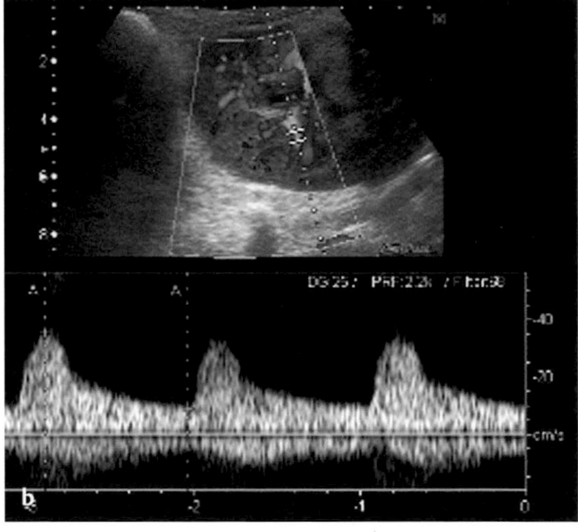

Resistance and pulsatility indices after renal transplant

Index	Formula	Normal range
Resistance index (RI)	$(V_{max} - V_{min})/V_{max}$	0.55 – 0.80
Pulsatility index (PI)	$(V_{max} - V_{min})/V_{mean}$	1.12 – 1.26

Selected References

Fischer T et al. A new method for standardized diagnosis following renal transplantation. Ultrasound with contrast enhancement. Urologe A 2006; 45: 38–45

Pozniak MA et al. Ultrasonographic evaluation of renal transplantation. Radiol Clin North Am 1992; 30: 1053–1066

Tanaka T et al. Correlation between the Banff 97 classification of renal allograft biopsies and clinical outcome. Transpl Int 2004; 17: 59–64

Imaging Signs

Surgical and nephrologic complications after kidney transplant.

- **Modality of choice**
  Ultrasound.
- **Ultrasound findings**
  Surgical complications:
  - Lymphocele or urinoma: Anechoic • Smoothly demarcated • Lymphocele may have septa.
  - Hematoma: Hypoechoic • Internal echoes may be present, depending on the degree of organization.
  - Ureteral obstruction/stricture: Hydronephrosis.
  - Arterial stenosis: TRAS is diagnosed if peak systolic velocity at the site of arterial anastomosis is increased above 190 cm/s and parenchymal RI is decreased
  - Venous thrombosis: Characteristic arterial flow curve with increased peak systolic velocity and end-diastolic flow reversal in combination with an increase in graft volume.
  - Pseudoaneurysm at the anastomotic site.
  - Arteriovenous fistula after core biopsy: will close spontaneously in most cases.

  Nephrologic complications:
  - Acute tubular necrosis: Reduced corticomedullary differentiation • Increased graft volume due to edema • Steep increase in RI (up to 1.0) and PI.
  - Acute rejection: Morphologic appearance does not allow reliable differentiation from acute tubular necrosis • Acute rejection may be suggested if graft volume increases by over 20% • Blurred corticomedullary junction • RI increase • Steep PI increase indicates acute tubular necrosis combined with acute rejection • Power Doppler ultrasound shows a wider unperfused peripheral margin.
  - Chronic rejection: Reduced peripheral perfusion (best appreciated by determining the unperfused peripheral margin using power Doppler ultrasound, “gnarled tree” sign may be seen).
- **MRI findings**
  - *Urinoma/lymphocele:* Well-defined lesion with high internal signal intensity on T2-weighted images • Hypointense fluid on T1-weighted images • Connection to the collecting system can be demonstrated by unenhanced MRI or MR IVP.
  - *Perirenal hematoma:* Low, intermediate, or high signal intensity depending on age of hemorrhage • Active bleeding will be demonstrated by MRA.
  - *Transplant renal artery stenosis:* Depicted as luminal narrowing on arterial phase MRA images.
  - *Transplant renal vein thrombosis:* Depicted as a filling defect in the dilated vein on venous phase MRA images.

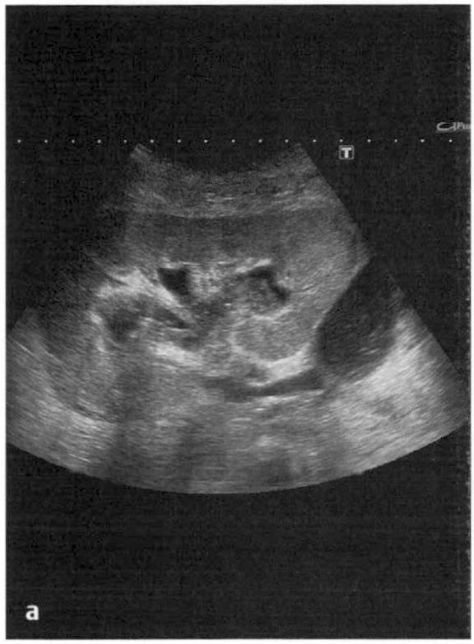

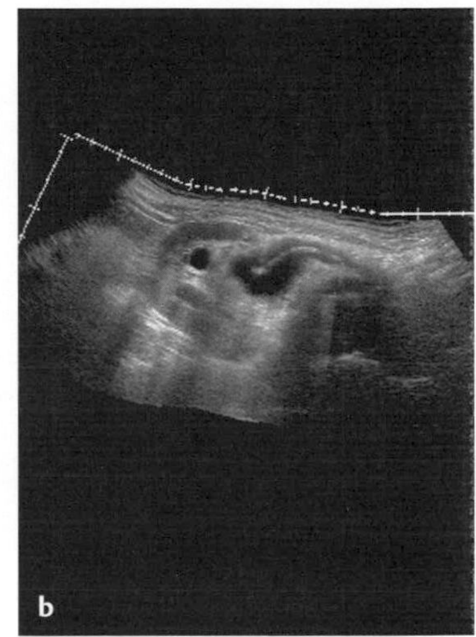

Fig. 1.42 a, b Lymphocele below the kidney graft (**a**). Ultrasound. Intermediate echogenicity indicates an increase in tissue around the ureteropelvic junction and proximal ureter (**b**). Ureteral stent. The appearance is consistent with chronic irritation.

▸ **CT**
CT is performed in patients with contraindications to MRI or on an emergency basis to detect active bleeding or acute transplant artery occlusion • Optimization of the contrast dose and saline flush before the scan is obtained.

▸ **Angiographic findings**
Direct demonstration of TRAS • PTA can be performed in the same session.

Clinical Aspects

▸ **Typical presentation**
Transplant renal vein thrombosis/TRAS is associated with hemorrhagic or ischemic graft infarction • New-onset renovascular hypertension • Increase in retention parameters • Hydronephrosis secondary to ureteral strictures or compression due to lymphocele/hematoma • No primary graft function in acute tubular necrosis.

▸ **Treatment options**
Treatment after confirmation of the diagnosis by graft biopsy • Immunosuppression • PTA of TRAS • Causal therapy of ureteral compression • Second transplant.

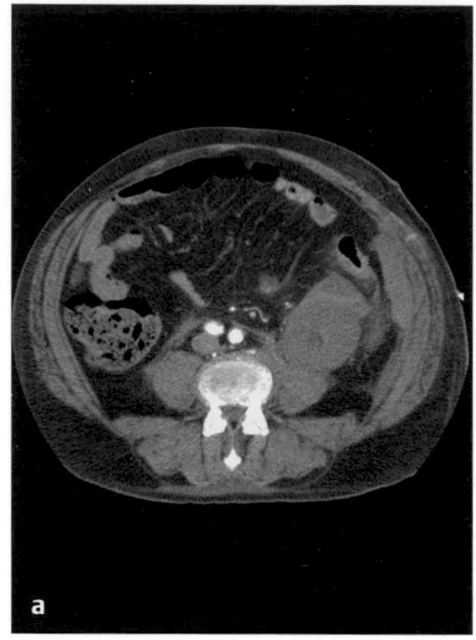
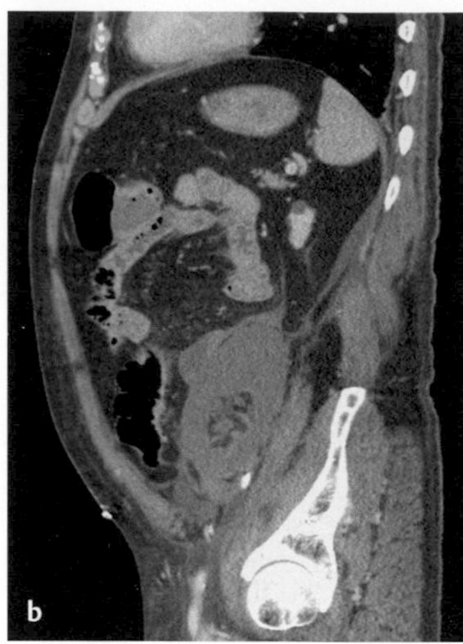

Fig. 1.43 a, b Acute occlusion of transplant renal artery and nonperfused ("silent") kidney graft. Biphasic multislice CT.
a Axial scan in the cortical phase.
b Sagittal MPR from the corticomedullary phase.

- **Course and prognosis**
  Characterization and staging of rejection episodes according to the Banff classification.
- **What does the clinical want to know?**
  Diagnosis • Relevance of complications.

Differential Diagnosis

Chronic CMV infection and cyclosporine toxicity	– These two entities must be considered in the differential diagnosis of acute tubular necrosis and rejection

Selected References

Pozniak MA et al. Ultrasonographic evaluation of renal transplantation. Radiol Clin North Am 1992; 30: 1053–1066

Tanaka T et al. Correlation between the Banff 97 classification of renal allograft biopsies and clinical outcome. Transpl Int 2004; 17: 59–64

Definition

Hyperplasia of the adrenal cortex typically affecting both glands • Diffuse hyperplasia is more common than nodular hyperplasia.

- **Epidemiology**
  Three to four times more common in men • Peak incidence in the third and fourth decades of life.
- **Etiology, pathophysiology**
  Often seen in Cushing syndrome (endogenous hypercortisolism) • Idiopathic bilateral adrenal cortex hyperplasia is rare • Dysregulation of the hypothalamus–pituitary–adrenal axis (ACTH-producing tumor of the anterior pituitary lobe, paraneoplasia, idiopathic) • Excessive cortisol production in functioning disease.

Imaging Signs

- **Modality of choice**
  MRI.
- **Pathognomonic findings**
  Bilateral enlargement of the adrenal glands with normal adreniform contour.
- **MRI findings**
  Normal adreniform shape with homogeneous or nodular enlargement of one or both adrenal limbs (> 10 mm) • Nearly isointense to muscle on T1-weighted images • Hyperintense to muscle on T2-weighted images • Typically both adrenals are affected; unilateral hyperplasia is very uncommon.
- **CT findings**
  Hypodense thickening of one or both adrenal limbs (> 10 mm).

Clinical Aspects

- **Typical presentation**
  Often asymptomatic and detected incidentally • Patients with functioning disease present with changes caused by hypercortisolism—moon face, truncal obesity, and buffalo hump due to abnormal accumulation of fat pads; hypertension.
- **Treatment options**
  Asymptomatic patients only need follow-up • Symptomatic patients are treated medically (bilateral involvement) or surgically (unilateral involvement).
- **Course and prognosis**
  Most patients respond well to medical treatment • Left untreated, Cushing syndrome is associated with high mortality.
- **What does the clinician want to know?**
  Unilateral or bilateral adrenocortical hyperplasia • Circumscribed mass visible?

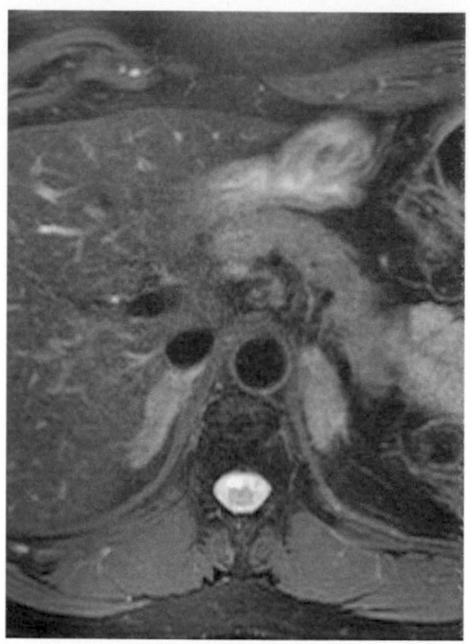

Fig. 1.44 Bilateral adrenocortical hyperplasia. Respiratory-triggered T2-weighted TSE MR image with fat saturation. Normal adreniform shape with thickening of the adrenal limbs. The signal intensity of the adrenals is higher than that of muscle.

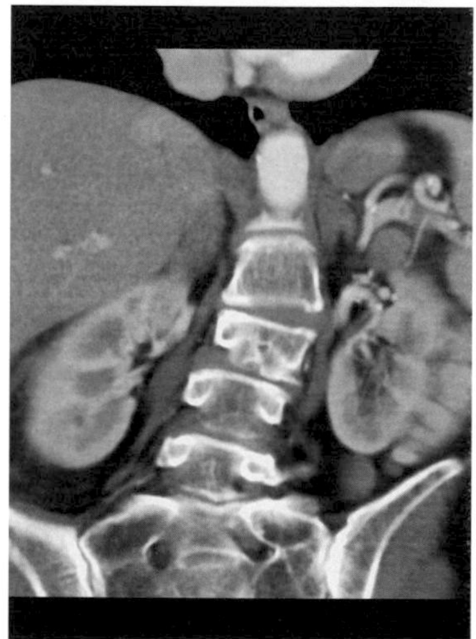

Fig. 1.45 Bilateral adrenocortical hyperplasia. Coronal reconstruction from CT data. Enlarged, hypodense adrenal glands.

Differential Diagnosis

Adenoma	– Circumscribed mass (or multiple masses) in an otherwise normal-sized adrenal gland – Homogeneous signal dropout on opposed-phase MR images (fat content)
Metastasis	– Focal lesion with strong contrast enhancement in an otherwise normal-sized adrenal gland

Selected References

Elsayes KM et al. Adrenal masses: MR imaging features with pathological correlation. Radiographics 2004; 24: S73–S86

Rockall AG et al. CT and MR imaging of the adrenal glands in ACTH-independent Cushing syndrome. Radiographics 2004; 24: 435–452

Definition

- **Epidemiology**
  Most common adrenal tumor • Prevalence increases with age • Up to 5% are incidentalomas on CT scans • *Size:* 0.5–10 cm; 50% smaller than 2 cm • 70% lipid-rich, 30% lipid-poor • Bilateral in 10% of cases • Adrenal adenomas are found in 10% of patients with Cushing syndrome, 75% of patients with Conn syndrome, and 80% with acquired adrenogenital syndrome.

Imaging Signs

- **Modality of choice**
  CT • MRI.
- **Pathognomonic findings**
  Diagnostic criteria:
  - Attenuation on unenhanced CT < 10 HU and size < 3 cm

  or
  - Washout on contrast-enhanced CT > 60%, relative washout > 40%, attenuation < 35 HU after 15 min, and size < 3 cm

  or
  - Signal decrease on MRI > 20% and size < 3 cm.

  Biopsy to resolve unclear cases.
- **CT findings**
  Sharply demarcated, homogeneous mass in the adrenal gland • Round to oval in shape • Typically less than 2 cm in size • No growth over 6 months • Calcification, hemorrhage, and necrosis are uncommon and mostly occur in large adenomas • Conn and Cushing adenomas are usually small at diagnosis because they cause symptoms related to hormone production • Atrophy of surrounding adrenal tissue and of contralateral gland • Morphologic appearance does not allow differentiation of functioning and nonfunctioning adenomas.
  Attenuation: Less than that of liver:
  - < 0 HU: 47% sensitivity, 100% specificity.
  - < 10 HU: 71% sensitivity, 98% specificity.
  - < 20 HU: 88% sensitivity, 84% specificity.

  Contrast enhancement pattern: Homogeneous, mild to moderate enhancement with rapid washout:
  - Washout: $HU_{60\,s}–HU_{15\,min}/HU_{60\,s}–HU_{pre} \times 100\% > 60\%$ (88% sensitivity, 96% specificity).
  - Relative washout: $HU_{60\,s}–HU_{15\,min}/HU_{60\,s} \times 100\% > 40\%$ (96% sensitivity, 100% specificity).

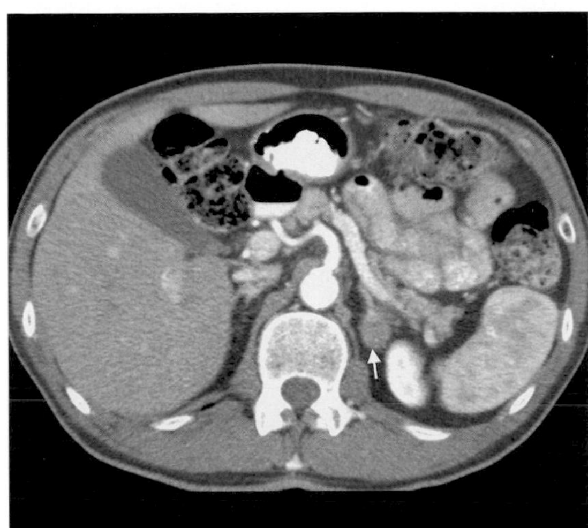

Fig. 1.46 Nonfunctioning adenoma (incidentaloma, arrow) in the left adrenal gland. Postcontrast CT scan shows slight enhancement of the mass.

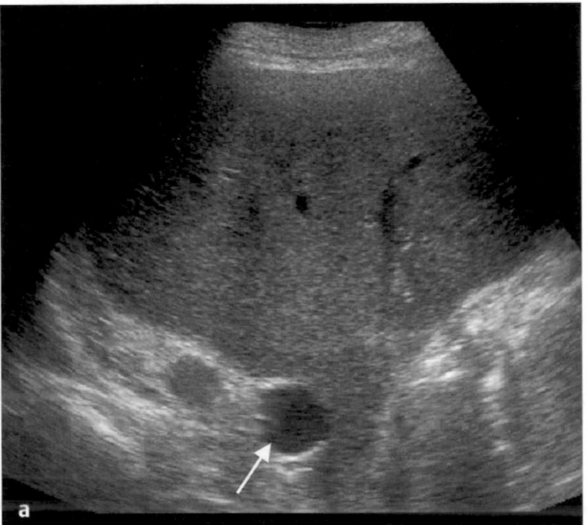

Fig. 1.47 a–c Right adrenal adenoma.

a Subcostal transheptic ultrasound view. Rounded hypoechoic mass. Arrow indicates the inferior vena cava medial to the lesion.

b Axial in-phase GRE MR image. Intermediate signal intensity of the adenoma (arrow).

c Axial opposed-phase GRE MR image. Pronounced signal dropout (arrow).

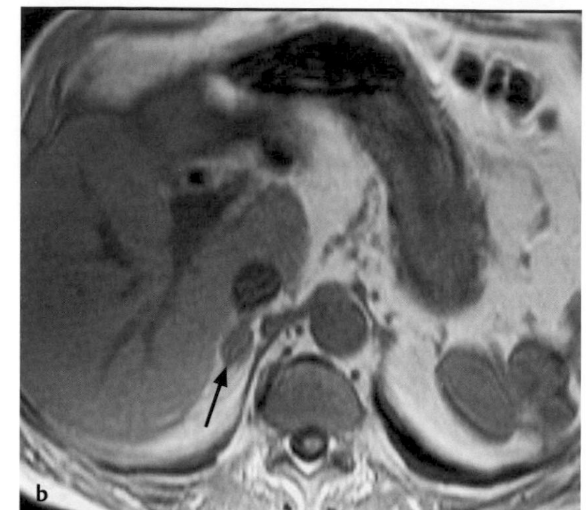

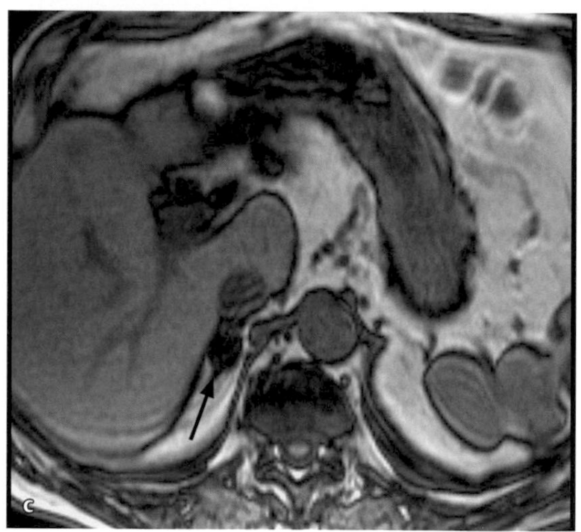

▸ **MRI findings**
Homogeneous mass in one adrenal gland • Isointense or hypointense to normal adrenal tissue and liver on T1- and T2-weighted images • Functioning adenoma has higher signal intensity on T2-weighted images • Homogeneous contrast enhancement • An occasional adenoma may contain small cystic areas or focal hemorrhage • Calcifications are rare • Chemical shift imaging for lipid detection—marked signal dropout on opposed-phase GRE images compared with in-phase GRE images:

- $SI_{opposed\text{-}phase}$ of lesion/$SI_{opposed\text{-}phase}$ of spleen/$SI_{in\text{-}phase}$ of lesion/$SI_{in\text{-}phase}$ of spleen × 100% < 70% (80–90% sensitivity, 100% specificity).
- $SI_{opposed\text{-}phase}$ of lesion/$SI_{in\text{-}phase}$ of lesion × 100% > 20%.

▸ **PET findings**
No increase in FDG uptake.

Clinical Aspects

▸ **Typical presentation**
Asymptomatic incidentaloma on CT scans obtained for other indications • Endocrinopathy in patients with functioning adrenal adenoma—hyperkalemic hypertension (Conn syndrome), excessive androgen secretion (adrenogenital syndrome).

▸ **Treatment options**
Treatment only in functioning adrenal adenoma—tumor resection and temporary hormone replacement in patients with suppressed adrenal function.

▸ **What does the clinician want to know?**
Confirmation of the diagnosis and exclusion of adrenal malignancy.

Differential Diagnosis

Macronodular hyperplasia	– Lobulated enlargement of the entire adrenal gland
Granulomatous adrenal inflammation	– Often bilateral – Low signal intensity on T1-weighted images and high signal intensity on T2-weighted images – Hyperintensities due to necrotic areas and signal voids due to calcifications on T2-weighted images – Contrast enhancement varies with the stage – Adrenal failure may ensue, especially in patients with histoplasmosis
Adrenal carcinoma/adrenal metastasis	– Larger and more heterogeneous – Rapid enhancement and slow washout – Higher signal intensity on T2-weighted images – Contain no fat

Pseudotumor	– Stomach, small intestine, diverticulum; oral contrast for differentiation – Accessory spleen or prominent splenic lobulation—smoothly marginated, same contrast enhancement pattern as the spleen – Vessels—contrast enhancement, signal loss on SE images
Myelolipoma	– Rare, benign, bilateral in 10% of cases – Typically 1–2 cm in size – Composed of mature adipose tissue with an attenuation of –10 HU – High signal intensity on T1- and T2-weighted images – Variable amount of soft tissue, nonfunctional tumor – Hemorrhage, necrosis, and calcification may be present
Ganglioneuroma	– Benign tumor – Oval lesion with smooth margins – Size and attenuation similar to those of adrenocortical carcinoma, therefore requiring biopsy
Mesenchymal adrenal tumors	– Very rare – Fibroma—low signal intensity – Lipoma—high signal intensity on T1-weighted images – Hemangioma—peripheral nodular enhancement with centripetal progression

Tips and Pitfalls

Make sure to differentiate a left adrenal mass from an accessory spleen.

Selected References

Elsayes KM et al. Adrenal masses: MR imaging features with pathologic correlation. RadioGraphics 2004; 24 (Suppl. 1): 73–86

Galanski M. Adrenal glands. In: Prokop M, Galanski M (eds). Computed Tomography of the Body. Stuttgart: Thieme; 2003

Mayo-Smith WW et al. State-of-the-art adrenal imaging. RadioGraphics 2001; 21: 995–1012

Definition

- **Epidemiology**

  Rare tumor • 1 case per 1 million • 50% have endocrine activity • Adrenocortical carcinoma occurs in 10% of patients with Cushing syndrome and 20% of patients with acquired adrenogenital syndrome.

Imaging Signs

- **Modality of choice**

  CT • MRI.
- **CT findings**

  Large adrenal mass (typically > 5 cm) • Heterogeneous appearance due to necrotic areas and hemorrhage • Irregular calcifications in 30% of tumors • Fatty foci are rare • Heterogeneous and rapid contrast enhancement, often sparing the necrotic center • Delayed washout • Tumor thrombus in the renal vein or inferior vena cava • Deformity and displacement of adjacent organs • Advanced carcinoma invades adjacent organs such as the liver, bones, and lungs • Metastatic spread to regional lymph nodes.
- **MRI findings**

  Large heterogeneous mass (typically > 5 cm) in one adrenal gland • Low signal intensity on T1-weighted images • High signal intensity on T2-weighted images, more than 3.5 times higher than that of muscle • *Hemorrhage:* High signal on T1-weighted images • *Postcontrast:* Marked, heterogeneous enhancement of the tumor without enhancement of the central necrosis; long plateau phase and delayed washout • Nonfunctioning adrenocortical carcinomas do not lose signal intensity on opposed-phase GRE images (difference < 5%) • Small carcinomas are homogeneous with high signal intensity on T2-weighted images with rapid, homogeneous enhancement after contrast administration.

Clinical Aspects

- **Typical presentation**

  May manifest as a hyperfunctioning mass causing Cushing syndrome in 35%, Cushing syndrome with virilization in 20%, virilization in 20%, and feminization in 5% • Risk of pulmonary artery embolism due to vascular thrombus.
- **Treatment options**

  Complete surgical resection, adjuvant radiotherapy, and adrenostatic therapy (mitotane) with simultaneous hormone replacement • Alternative option: chemotherapy.
- **Prognosis**

  Very poor.
- **What does the clinician want to know?**

  Differentiation from benign adrenal tumors • Staging.

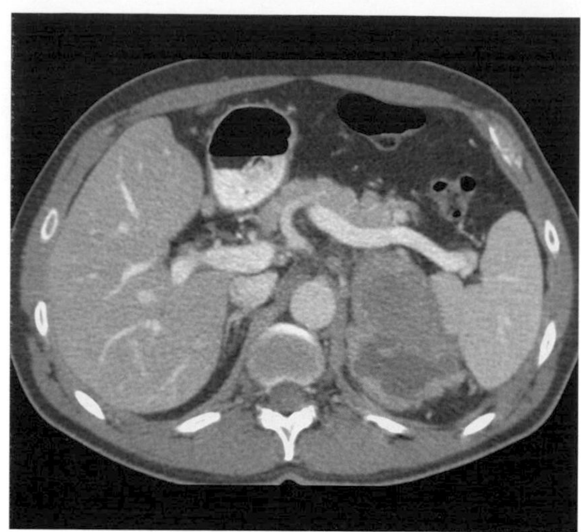

Fig. 1.48 Large adrenocortical carcinoma in the left adrenal gland of a 61-year-old patient who presented with back pain and raised blood pressure. Contrast-enhanced CT scan showing heterogeneous attenuation. Histologic examination demonstrated no extracapsular extension.

Differential Diagnosis

Adrenal metastasis
- No reliable differentiation based on morphology
- More common than primary adrenocortical carcinoma
- Often 2–3 cm in size, may occur in both glands
- History

Pheochromocytoma
- Radiomorphologic criteria do not always allow differentiation
- Heterogeneous, large, 10% affect both glands
- 10% of pheochromocytomas are malignant
- Blood chemistry and clinical findings point to the diagnosis

Malignant lymphoma
- No reliable differentiation based on morphology
- Mostly in patients with NHL
- Bilateral in 50% of cases
- Concomitant enlargement of retroperitoneal lymph nodes is common
- High signal intensity on T2-weighted images, long plateau phase after contrast administration

Adrenal adenoma
- Very large adenomas with regressive changes are rare
- Contains fat

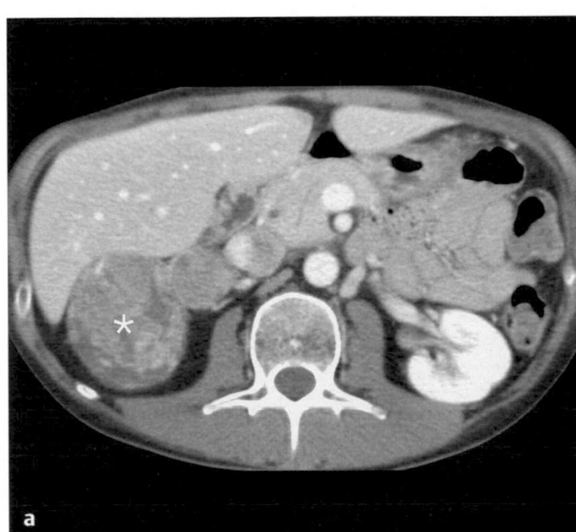

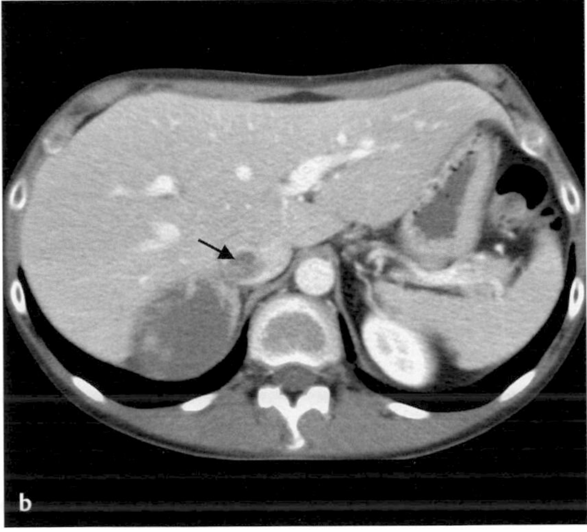

Fig. 1.49 a, b Cortisol-producing carcinoma in the cortex (asterisk in **a**) of the right adrenal gland in a 29-year-old patient with symptoms of Cushing syndrome. Contrast-enhanced CT. Heterogeneous attenuation. Tumor extending into the inferior vena cava (arrow in **b**). Histologic examination demonstrated extraadrenal tumor extension into surrounding fatty tissue. Pulmonary metastases were already present at diagnosis.

Neuroblastoma	– Most common malignant abdominal tumor under 5 years of age – Arises from the sympathetic ganglia or adrenal medulla – Heterogeneous appearance due to necrosis, hemorrhage, and cysts; often calcified; low signal on T1-weighted images and high signal on T2-weighted images – Marked contrast enhancement – Tendency towards extraglandular tumor extension, metastatic spread, and paraneoplasia
Ganglioneuroma	– Size and attenuation similar to those of adrenocortical carcinoma; biopsy – Benign tumor of sympathetic origin – Ganglioneuroma of the adrenal cortex typically at age 30–50
Ganglioneuroblastoma	– Most often in infants and children up to 10 years of age – Often retroperitoneal – Ganglioneuroblastoma of the adrenal cortex is a small tumor with smooth margins, less malignant than a neuroblastoma, and often calcified – Moderate, heterogeneous contrast enhancement – Regional lymph node metastases

Selected References

Elsayes KM et al. Adrenal masses: MR imaging features with pathologic correlation. RadioGraphics 2004; 24 (Suppl. 1): 73–86

Mayo-Smith WW et al. State-of-the-art adrenal imaging. RadioGraphics 2001; 21: 995–1012

Prokop M, Galanski M. Adrenal glands. In: Prokop M, Galanski M (eds). Computed Tomography of the Body. Stuttgart: Thieme; 2003

Definition

- **Epidemiology**
  Though rare, pheochromocytoma is the most common tumor of the adrenal medulla • 10% are malignant • 10% are bilateral • 10% are extra-adrenal or ectopic (paraganglioma) • 80% produce epinephrine, 20% norepinephrine • 10% are familial—MEN (usually bilateral, intraadrenal, and multiple), neurofibromatosis, von Hippel–Lindau disease.

Imaging Signs

- **Modality of choice**
  MRI • Nuclear medicine imaging.
- **MRI findings**
  Pheochromocytoma has low signal intensity on T1-weighted images and high signal intensity on T2-weighted images • Strong contrast enhancement • Intralesional hemorrhage, central necrosis, and multiple cysts are common • 10% show calcifications • Paraganglioma has high signal intensity on T2-weighted images • Recurrent pheochromocytoma after resection has high signal intensity on T2-weighted images.
- **Nuclear medicine imaging findings**
  ^{131}I-metaiodobenzylguanidine (norepinephrine analogue) or ^{111}In-octreotide (somatostatin analogue) for localizing ectopic pheochromocytoma • Whole-body scan 24–72 hours after nuclide administration.
- **CT findings**
  Adrenal pheochromocytoma is visualized as a smoothly marginated or irregular round mass • Typically > 3 cm in size • Often hemorrhagic, necrotic, cystic, and calcified • Attenuation of small tumors is homogeneous and similar to that of liver • *Paraganglioma:* Kidneys; retroperitoneum (typically at the aortic bifurcation); rarely in the mediastinum, gonads, urinary bladder • Multiple in 10% of cases (mostly in patients with MEN).

Clinical Aspects

- **Typical presentation**
  Paroxysmal or sustained hypertension and tachycardia • Headache.
- **Treatment options**
  Tumor resection • Perioperative α-adrenergic blockage and antihypertensive therapy • Catecholamine inhibitors (metyrosine) and chemotherapy in patients with unresectable pheochromocytoma.
- **Prognosis**
  Chronic cardiovascular disease in 25% of patients after resection • 5-year survival rate of 50% in patients with metastatic pheochromocytoma.
- **What does the clinician want to know?**
  Diagnosis • Differential diagnostic workup.

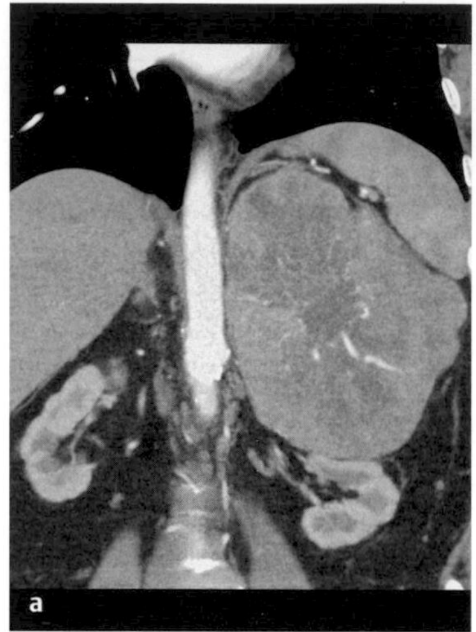

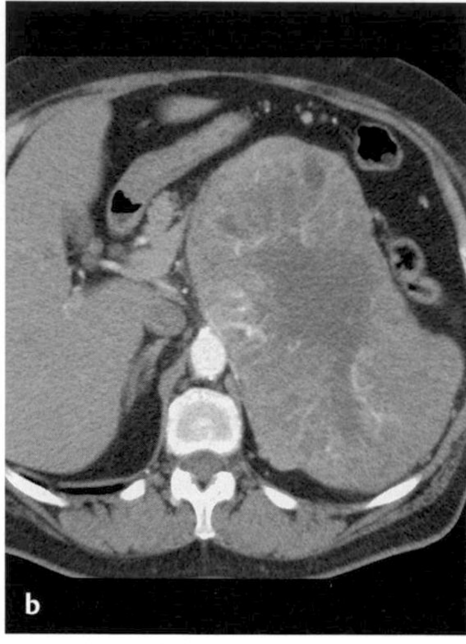

Fig. 1.50 a, b Large pheochromocytoma in the left adrenal gland of a 65-year-old patient. Coronal (**a**) and axial (**b**) CT scans after contrast administration. Heterogeneous attenuation, central necrosis, and radially arranged tumor vessels. Downward displacement of the left kidney and anterior displacement of the pancreas.

Differential Diagnosis

Adrenal metastasis	– History – Often bilateral – Nonfunctioning – Differential diagnosis cannot be made in all cases based on morphology and enhancement pattern
Adrenal carcinoma	– Less common – Unilateral – 50% are hyperfunctioning – Differential diagnosis cannot be made in all cases based on morphology and enhancement pattern
Neuroblastoma	– Most common malignant abdominal tumor in infants and children – 75% of neuroblastomas occur before the age of 2 years – Arises from the sympathetic ganglia or adrenal medulla – Large – Heterogeneous appearance due to necrosis and hemorrhage – Often tiny calcifications – Marked contrast enhancement – Invasion of surrounding tissues, early metastatic spread (bone, lymph nodes)
Adrenal cyst	– Small cyst with smooth walls

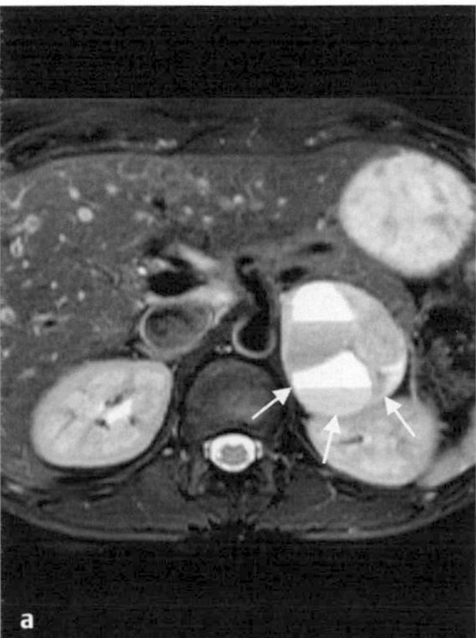

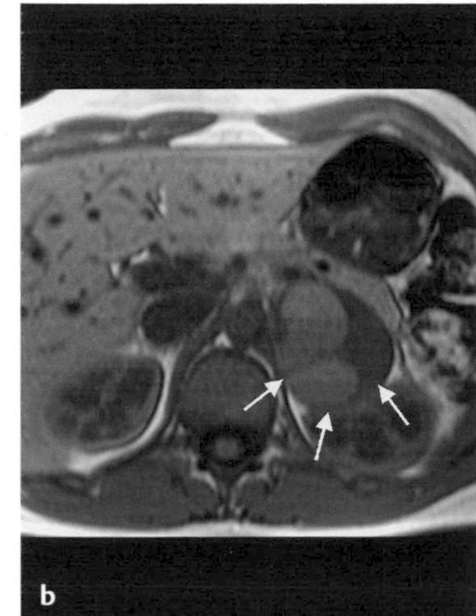

Fig. 1.51 a, b Pheochromocytoma (arrows) in the left adrenal gland of a 35-year-old patient with hypertensive episodes. Axial T2-weighted (**a**) and T1-weighted (**b**) MR images. Intracystic hemorrhage with sedimentation produces fluid-debris levels within the cyst. Histologic examination revealed no extracapsular extension.

Tips and Pitfalls

Do not puncture the adrenals in patients with suspected pheochromocytoma (hypertensive crisis).

Selected References

Elsayes KM et al. Adrenal masses: MR imaging features with pathologic correlation. RadioGraphics 2004; 24 (Suppl. 1): 73–86

Mayo-Smith WW et al. State-of-the-art adrenal imaging. RadioGraphics 2001; 21: 995–1012

Prokop M, Galanski M. Adrenal glands. In: Prokop M, Galanski M (eds). Computed Tomography of the Body. Stuttgart: Thieme; 2003

Definition

- **Epidemiology**
  Most common malignancy of the adrenal glands in adults • Found at autopsy in 27% of cancer patients • Often bilateral.
- **Etiology**
  Most common primary tumors: Lung and breast tumors, malignant melanoma, renal cell carcinoma, pancreatic carcinoma • Pancreatic and renal cell carcinomas can invade the adrenals by direct contiguous extension.

Imaging Signs

- **Modality of choice**
  CT • MRI • PET.
- **CT findings**
  Large metastases: Heterogeneous, lobulated, irregular margin • Hemorrhage is common • Calcification is rare • Intratumoral cyst with thick, irregular, contrast-enhancing wall is uncommon • Heterogeneous contrast enhancement.
  Small metastases: < 3 cm, homogeneous, round, smoothly marginated masses that do not contain fat.
- **MRI findings**
  Low signal intensity on T1-weighted images, high signal intensity on T2-weighted images; less common adrenal metastases have signal characteristics similar to the primary • Large metastases are heterogeneous due to necrosis and hemorrhage • Small metastases are homogeneous • Pronounced contrast enhancement and delayed washout • No signal decrease on opposed-phase GRE images.
- **PET findings**
  Malignant adrenal tumors have higher FDG uptake than inflammatory lesions.

Clinical Aspects

- **Typical presentation**
  Most adrenal metastases are asymptomatic • Typically detected during staging or follow-up of cancer patients.
- **Treatment options**
  Depend on the primary tumor • Surgical resection with adjuvant chemotherapy or primary chemotherapy.
- **Prognosis**
  Depends on the primary tumor • Very poor.
- **What does the clinician want to know?**
  Differential diagnostic workup.

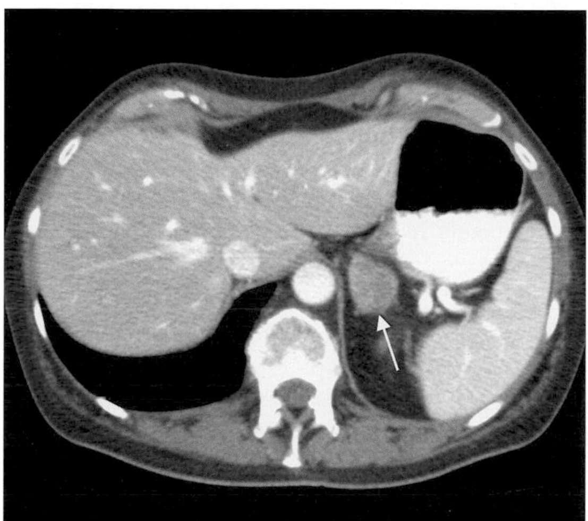

Fig. 1.52 Metastasis in the left adrenal gland (arrow) in a patient with metastatic malignant melanoma. CT after contrast administration.

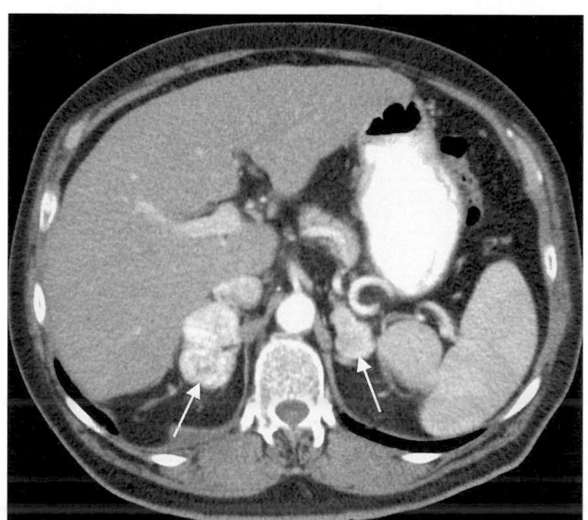

Fig. 1.53 Hypervascular metastases from renal cell carcinoma in both adrenal glands (arrows). CT after contrast administration.

Differential Diagnosis

Lipid-poor adenomas (30% of adrenal adenomas)	– Cannot be differentiated on the basis of their CT attenuation or MR signal intensity – Stronger washout
Adrenocortical carcinoma	– Rare, endocrine activity in 50% – Unilateral – Radiomorphologic criteria do not allow reliable differentiation
Pheochromocytoma	– Rare – May also occur bilaterally – Higher signal intensity on T2-weighted images but no reliable differentiation on the basis of radiomorphologic criteria alone – Differential diagnosis based on blood chemistry tests

Selected References

Elsayes KM et al. Adrenal masses: MR imaging features with pathologic correlation. RadioGraphics 2004; 24 (Suppl. 1): 73–86

Mayo-Smith WW et al. State-of-the-art adrenal imaging. RadioGraphics 2001; 21: 995–1012

Prokop M, Galanski M. Adrenal glands. In: Prokop M, Galanski M (eds). Computed Tomography of the Body. Stuttgart: Thieme; 2003

Definition

- **Etiology**
  Adrenal hemorrhage: Most common cause in children/neonates; in adults usually associated with trauma, typically of the right gland • Anticoagulant therapy, coagulopathy, burns, shock, surgery, septicemia (Waterhouse–Friderichsen syndrome) • Bilateral in 10–20% of cases.
  Granulomatous inflammation: Tuberculosis, histoplasmosis, sarcoidosis.

Imaging Signs

- **Modality of choice**
  CT.
- **CT findings**
  - *Calcification after hemorrhage:* Onset of calcification after 1 week in children and after about 1 year in adults • Eggshell calcification indicates pseudocyst • Atrophy.
  - *Acute hemorrhage:* Hyperdense adrenal mass (40–80 HU) • Imbibition of surrounding fatty tissue • No contrast enhancement.
  - *Calcification following infection:* Multiple calcifications of variable hyperdensity • Patchy appearance • Adrenal atrophy.
  - *Acute infection:* Symmetric and nodular enlargement of both adrenals • Hypodense granulomas • Peripheral contrast enhancement or heterogeneous enhancement if necrotic areas are present • Concomitant lymphadenopathy.
- **MRI findings**
  Calcifications are seen as signal voids on T1- and T2-weighted images •
  Hemorrhage: Adrenal enlargement and high signal intensity on T2-weighted images in the acute stage.
  Signal intensity of hematoma varies with age:
  - *Acute* (up to 7 days): Isointense on T1-weighted images, low signal intensity on T2-weighted images.
  - *Subacute* (up to 7 weeks): High signal intensity on T1-weighted images and increasing signal intensity on T2-weighted images.
  - *Chronic* (older than 7 weeks): High signal intensity on T1- and T2-weighted images.

Clinical Aspects

- **Typical presentation**
  Calcifications are usually asymptomatic • Acute hemorrhage can present with Addison crisis (shock, acute abdomen) • Addison disease when there is chronic destruction of over 90% of adrenal tissue (nonspecific weakness, nausea) • Nonspecific inflammatory symptoms of adrenal infection.
- **Treatment options**
  Calcifications do not require treatment • Hormone substitution in Addison disease.

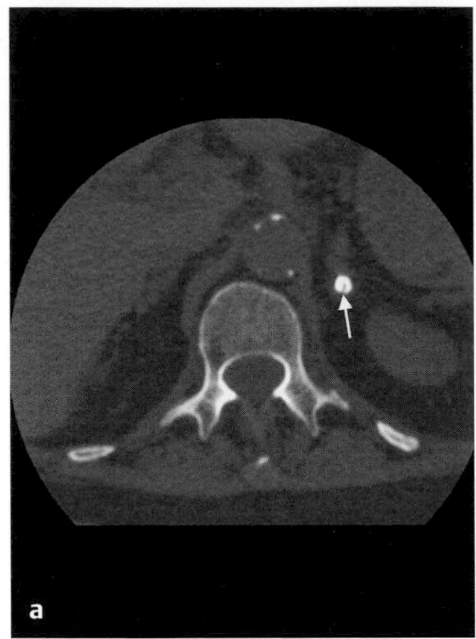

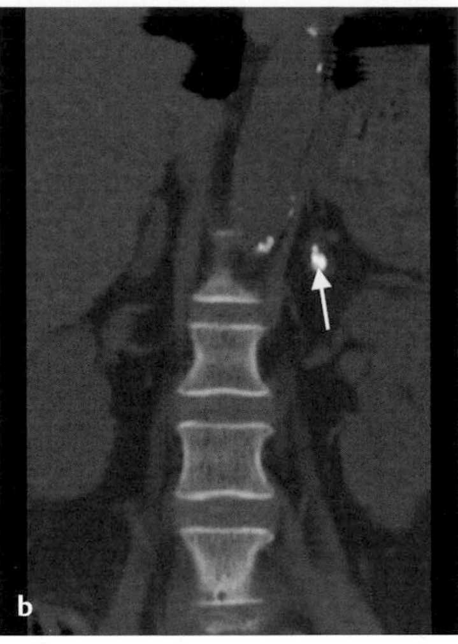

Fig. 1.54 a, b Adrenal calcification. Axial CT scan (**a**) and coronal reconstruction (**b**). Nodular enlargement of both adrenal glands. Punctate calcification in the left adrenal (arrows).

▸ **What does the clinician want to know?**
Differentiation from calcified adrenal tumor.

Differential Diagnosis

Calcified adrenal tumor	– Associated soft tissue mass – Calcifications in 80% of neuroblastomas, 30% of adrenal carcinomas, and 10% of pheochromocytomas – Diffuse and irregular distribution of calcifications
Addison disease of other etiology	– Autoimmune-induced (most common cause in industrialized countries) – Small adrenal glands or bilateral adrenal tumors

Selected References

Elsayes KM et al. Adrenal masses: MR imaging features with pathologic correlation. RadioGraphics 2004; 24 (Suppl. 1): 73–86

Federle MP et al. Diagnostic Imaging—Adomen. Amirsys; 2005

Mayo-Smith WW et al. From the RSNA refresher course: State-of-the-art adrenal imaging. RadioGraphics 2001; 21: 995–1012

Prokop M, Galanski M. Adrenal glands. In: Prokop M, Galanski M (eds). Computed Tomography of the Body. Stuttgart: Thieme; 2003

Definition

- **Epidemiology**
  Rare • May occur at any age • More common in women • Bilateral in 19% of cases • *Types of adrenal cysts:* 50% endothelial and epithelial cysts, 40% pseudocysts, and 10% parasitic cysts (echinococcal).
- **Etiology**
  Endothelial cysts are attributed by some to obstructed adrenal lymph vessels • Pseudocysts occur secondary to hemorrhage or cystic liquefaction.

Imaging Signs

- **Modality of choice**
  CT • Ultrasound • MRI.
- **CT findings**
  Smoothly marginated lesion • Thin cyst wall, up to 3 mm • Low attenuation of cyst fluid (0–20 HU) • Pseudocyst with septa and wall calcifications, fluid levels may be present • Echinococcal cyst with wall calcifications • No wall enhancement.
  Ultrasound findings
  Anechoic • Smoothly demarcated • Delicate wall.
- **MRI findings**
  Rounded adrenal mass • Smoothly delineated • Low signal intensity on T1-weighted images, high signal on T2-weighted images • No enhancement • Pseudocysts may contain blood components, septa, and soft tissue components • No increase in size.

Clinical Aspects

- **Typical presentation**
  Asymptomatic incidental finding • Acute pain due to hemorrhage is rare.
- **Treatment options**
  No treatment required.

Differential Diagnosis

Regressive adrenal carcinoma/ regressive adrenal metastasis	– Liquefied center and thicker, irregular wall – Typically higher attenuation than cyst fluid – Increase in size – Strong contrast enhancement of solid components
Cystic adenoma, adrenal carcinoma, pheochromocytoma, cystic lymphangioma	– Solid tumor component, visible in most cases – Increase in size

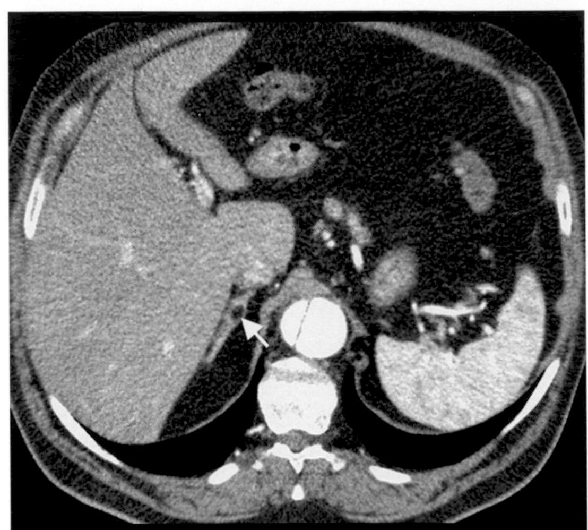

Fig. 1.55 Adrenal cyst. CT after contrast administration. Hypoattenuating cyst 11 mm in size (arrow) in the medial limb of the right adrenal gland. Incidental finding with unchanged appearance at follow-up. Accessory finding—dissection of the abdominal aorta.

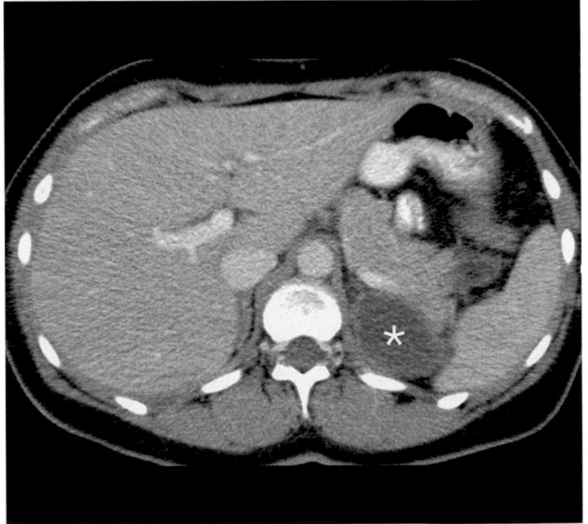

Fig. 1.56 Adrenal cyst. CT after contrast administration. Cyst 4 × 5 cm in size (asterisk) between the limbs of the left adrenal gland. Attenuation of the cyst content slightly more than that of water. An adrenal cyst was diagnosed after resection.

Selected References

Elsayes KM et al. Adrenal masses: MR imaging features with pathologic correlation. RadioGraphics 2004; 24 (Suppl. 1): 73–86

Mayo-Smith WW et al. State-of-the-art adrenal imaging. RadioGraphics 2001; 21: 995–1012

Prokop M, Galanski M. Adrenal glands. In: Prokop M, Galanski M (eds). Computed Tomography of the Body. Stuttgart: Thieme; 2003

Definition

Bifid ureter: A single distal ureter drains into the bladder through a single orifice • The common segment divides into two branches at a variable level to drain a duplicated collecting system.

Double ureter: Two completely separate ureters drain a duplicated collecting system • One of the two ureters inserts ectopically, usually inferior to the orthotopic orifice.

- **Etiology**
  Developmental • Usually a normal variant • Found on IVP in 6–8% of cases and affects more women than men • Bifid ureters may occasionally be associated with ureteroureteral reflux into the lower pelvicaliceal system or UPJ obstruction of the lower pole moiety • Double ureters are frequently associated with VUR and occasionally with ectopic ureterocele.

Imaging Signs

- **Modality of choice**
  IVP.
- **Pathognomonic findings**
  Elongated kidney with a duplicated collecting system and ureter.
- **Intravenous pyelogram findings**
  The pelvicaliceal system of the upper pole moiety is usually smaller • When duplicated ureters insert separately into the bladder, the upper pole ureter drains below the lower pole ureter (Weigert–Meyer rule).
  Ectopic ureteral orifice: Ureter empties more inferiorly and medially into the bladder • May occasionally insert into the prostatic urethra in men/into the vagina or urethra in women.
- **Ultrasound findings**
  Duplex kidney often longer than normal kidney • Duplication of the collecting system and ureter.
- **Voiding cystourethrography findings**
  VUR is more commonly found in patients with double ureter, less commonly in bifid ureter.
- **MRI findings**
  Exact anatomic position of the ectopic ureteral orifice and course of the ureter through the pelvis.

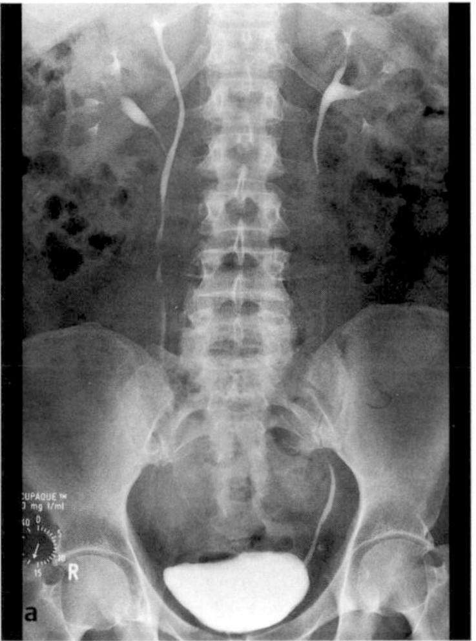

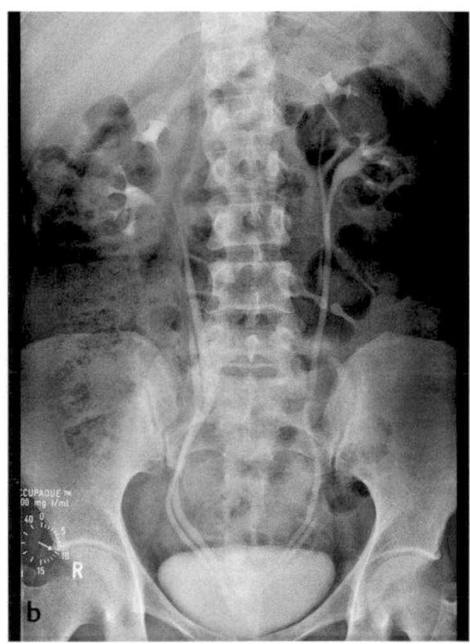

Fig. 2.1 a, b Anomalies of the ureter. IVP.
a High bifid ureter on the right side.
b Double ureter on both sides.

Clinical Aspects

- **Typical presentation**
  - *Bifid ureter:* Asymptomatic in most cases • Recurrent UTI if associated with obstruction or VUR.
  - *Double ureter:* Recurrent UTI is more common and is more often due to reflux.
  - *Ectopic insertion outside the bladder:* Nycturia • Recurrent UTI • Urinary incontinence (especially in women).
- **Treatment options**
  Treatment only in the presence of reflux or obstruction • *Medical treatment:* Antibiotics in case of infection • *Surgery:* Reimplantation of the ectopic ureter, which may be combined with resection of the atrophic moiety.
- **Prognosis**
  Good in most cases • Depends on the severity of renal damage caused by reflux or obstruction.
- **What does the clinician want to know?**
  Exact characterization of the anomaly.

Differential Diagnosis

Crossed renal ectopia	– Two kidneys on one side of the body – No kidney on the other side – Two crossed ureters that insert orthotopically

Tips and Pitfalls

The upper pole moiety in patients with double ureter is often the target of recurrent infection but may be missed by IVP because it is atrophic and does not excrete contrast.

Selected References

Berrocal T et al. Anomalies of the distal ureter, bladder, and urethra in children: embryologic, radiologic and pathologic features. Radiographics 2002; 22: 1139–1164

Bisset GS 3rd, Strife JL. The duplex collecting system in girls with urinary tract infection: prevalence and significance. AJR Am J Roentgenol 1987; 148: 497–500

Fernbach SK et al. Ureteral duplication and its complications. Radiographics 1997; 17: 109–127

Definition

- **Etiology**
  Enlargement of the ureter typically in association with dilatation of the pelvicaliceal system. Primary megaureter due to a developmental abnormality.
  - *Primary obstructive megaureter (ureteral achalasia):* Due to an ectopic aperistaltic segment of the distal ureter that cannot propagate urine properly.
  - *Primary refluxing megaureter:* Secondary to VUR.
  - *Secondary megaureter:* Obstruction at the level of the bladder or urethra (neurogenic bladder, urethral valve).

Imaging Signs

- **Modality of choice**
  MRI • Ultrasound.
- **Pathognomonic findings**
  Massive dilatation of the ureter that is most pronounced just above the bladder.
- **MRI findings**
  Aperistaltic segment • Ureteral dilatation increases from top to bottom.
- **Ultrasound findings**
  Normal antegrade and abnormal retrograde peristaltic waves of the dilated ureter.
- **Intravenous pyelogram findings**
  Enlargement of the ureter (diameter > 7 mm) with prominent dilatation just above the urinary bladder • Dilated portion funnels into the aperistaltic segment (not with primary refluxing and secondary megaureter).
- **Voiding cystourethrography findings**
  VCUG necessary to exclude reflux • Will identify ureteral dilatation only in primary refluxing megaureter.

Clinical Aspects

- **Typical presentation**
  Recurrent UTI.
- **Treatment options**
  - *Primary obstructive megaureter:* Resection of the aperistaltic segment.
  - *Primary refluxing megaureter:* Conservative • 50% spontaneous resolution rate.
  - *Secondary megaureter:* Relief of underlying obstruction.
- **Course and prognosis**
  Depend on secondary renal damage.
- **What does the clinician want to know?**
  Differentiation of obstructive and refluxing megaureter • Concomitant anomalies.

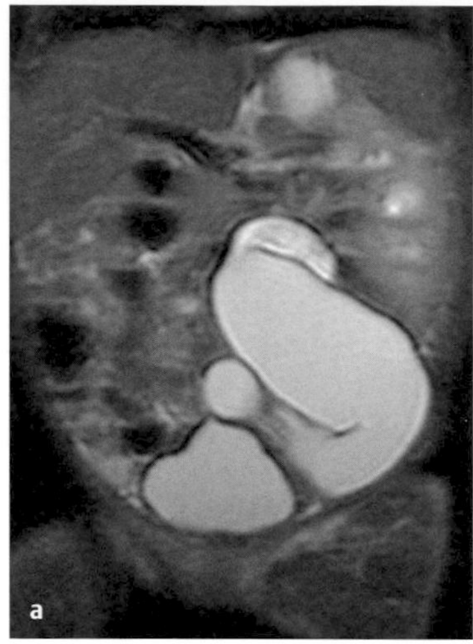

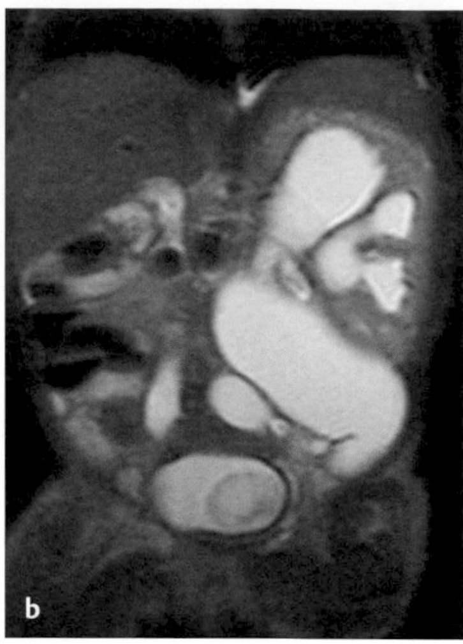

Fig. 2.2 a, b Megaureter on the left in a child. Coronal T2-weighted single-shot TSE MR images. There is massive enlargement of the left ureter throughout its course (**a, b**) with concomitant marked dilatation of the ipsilateral pelvicaliceal system (**b**).

Differential Diagnosis

Distal urinary obstruction – Cause can be directly identified (tumor, calculus)

Tips and Pitfalls

The aperistaltic segment may be overlooked because it may dilate slightly if only a retrograde pyelogram is obtained.

Selected References

Berrocal T et al. Anomalies of the distal ureter, bladder, and urethra in children: embryologic, radiologic and pathologic features. Radiographics 2002; 22: 1139–1164

Liu HY et al. Clinical outcome and management of prenatally diagnosed primary megaureters. J Urol 1994; 152: 614–617

Wilcox D, Mouriquand P. Management of megaureter in children. Eur Urol 1998; 34: 73–78

Definition

Spherical protrusion of the intramural ureter into the lumen of the urinary bladder.

- **Epidemiology, etiology**
  Developmental abnormality • Dilatation of the distal ureter and protrusion into the bladder lumen often result from congenital stricture of the intramural ureteral segment • More common in women • 75% of patients have concomitant double ureter • Can cause secondary megaureter.

Imaging Signs

- **Modality of choice**
  IVP, ultrasound (especially in children).
- **Pathognomonic findings**
  Cobra head appearance (see below).
- **Intravenous pyelogram findings**
  Collection of contrast medium surrounded by a radiolucent line (the typical cobra head appearance) within the bladder • Located at the ureteral orifice • Best appreciated 10 minutes after contrast administration • Often associated with urinary obstruction • Possible megaureter.
- **Ultrasound findings**
  Anechoic mass protruding into the bladder lumen • Smooth outline • Contiguous with the ureter, which is often dilated.

Clinical Aspects

- **Typical presentation**
  Usually asymptomatic in adults • Obstruction in children (often diagnosed prenatally) • Recurrent UTI due to VUR.
- **Treatment options**
  No intervention in adults and in the absence of symptoms • Resection in children, especially when complications are present (infection, calculus formation, obstruction, hydronephrosis).
- **What does the clinician want to know?**
  Concomitant anomalies: Multicystic dysplastic kidney, hydronephrosis (nearly always affecting the upper pole moiety in patients with duplex kidney).

Differential Diagnosis

Urothelial carcinoma at the UVJ	– Irregular outline – Thickened wall on ultrasound
Seminal vesicle cyst	– Multicystic structure – Inhomogeneous internal structure
Paraureteral bladder diverticulum	– Becomes visible only when the bladder is filled – Neck will be seen on lateral projections

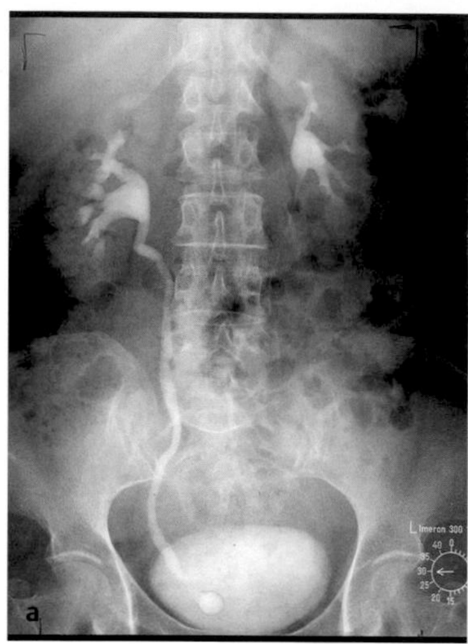

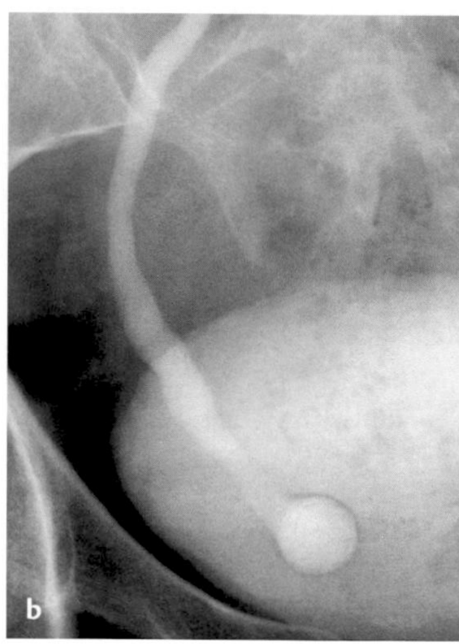

Fig. 2.3 a, b Ureterocele on the right. IVP.

a Rounded collection of contrast medium surrounded by a thin radiolucent line (cobra head) in the area of the right UVJ. Urinary obstruction is indicated by opacification and slight dilatation of the entire ipsilateral ureter. The calices of the right kidney are splayed.

b Magnified view with good visualization of the radiolucent line.

Tips and Pitfalls

If the first IVP film after contrast administration is obtained too late, a ureterocele may be missed because it is compressed by the increasing bladder filling pressure or obscured by contrast in the bladder.

Selected References

Berrocal T et al. Anomalies of the distal ureter, bladder, and urethra in children: embryologic, radiologic and pathologic features. Radiographics 2002; 22: 1139–1164

Karmazyn B, Zerin JM. Lower urinary tract abnormalities in children with multicystic dysplastic kidney. Radiology 1997; 203: 223–226

Zerin JM, Baker DR, Casale JA. Single-system ureteroceles in infants and children: imaging features. Pediatr Radiol 2000; 30: 139–146

Definition

Anomalies causing urinary obstruction at the anatomic junction of the renal pelvis and ureter with subsequent hydronephrosis.

- **Etiology**
  Congenital developmental anomaly • Five times more common in men • Predominantly caused by an accessory/aberrant vessel compressing the UPJ • Congenital stenosis of the UPJ • High ureteral insertion into the renal pelvis.

Imaging Signs

- **Modality of choice**
  MRI with MRA.
- **Pathognomonic findings**
  Ballooning of the pelvicaliceal system with little or no opacification of the ureter.
- **MRI and CT findings**
  Downward distention or ballooning of the pelvicaliceal system • Persistent nephrogram • Cause of obstruction (vessel) may be seen directly.
- **Intravenous pyelogram findings**
  Downward distention or ballooning of the pelvicaliceal system • Poor or no opacification of the ureter • Persistent nephrogram.
- **Ultrasound findings**
  Anechoic, massively dilated pelvicaliceal system • Parenchymal thinning.

Clinical Aspects

- **Typical presentation**
  Often asymptomatic • Intermittent flank pain, can be provoked by large fluid intake.
- **Treatment options**
  Surgical repair by pyeloplasty or vascular intervention.
- **Course and prognosis**
  Depend on whether there is loss of renal function at presentation • If yes, prompt treatment is required to prevent further progression and irreversible renal damage.
- **What does the clinician want to know?**
  Presence of an underlying anatomic cause.

Differential Diagnosis

Acquired obstruction	– Calculus – Tumor – Compression by aneurysm

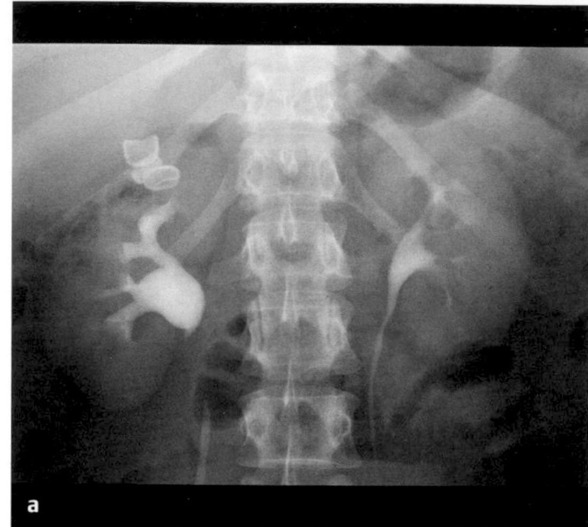

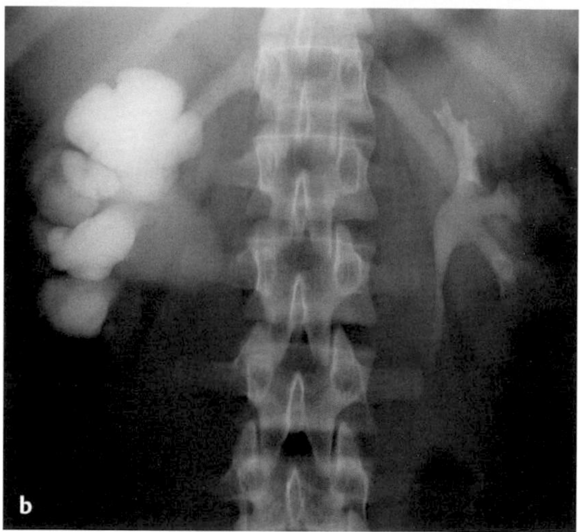

Fig. 2.4 a, b Congenital UPJ stenoses causing various degrees of urinary obstruction. IVP.

a Downward distention of the right renal pelvis. The pelvis tapers into the ureter and there is only mild outflow obstruction. Accessory finding: gallstones.

b Highest-grade stenosis of the right UPJ. Ballooning of the pelvicaliceal system.

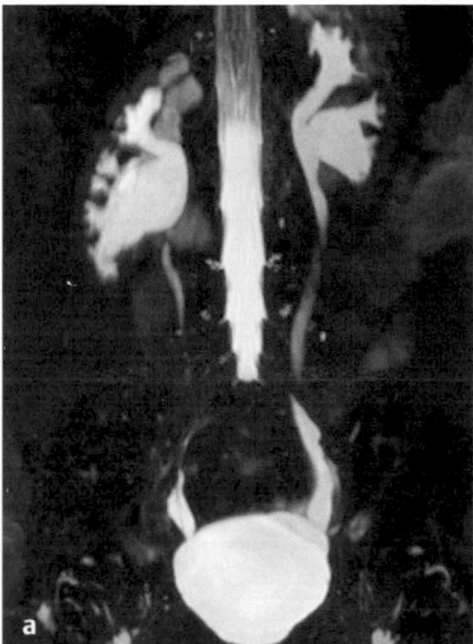

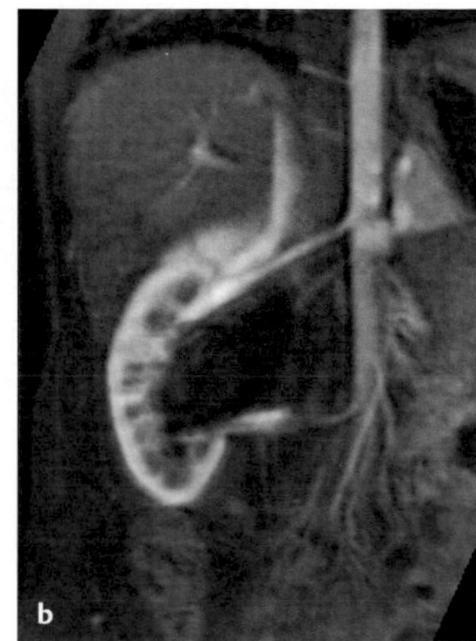

Fig. 2.5 a, b Compression of the UPJ by an accessory renal artery.
a MIP reconstructed from a stack of T2-weighted TSE MR images. Dilated collecting system and downward distention of the right renal pelvis.
b MRA showing the accessory renal artery.

Tips and Pitfalls

A small accessory artery overlooked during preoperative diagnostic workup can lead to intraoperative bleeding.

Selected References

Lawler LP et al. Adult ureteropelvic junction obstruction: insights with three-dimensional multi-detector row CT. Radiographics 2005; 25: 121–134

Siegel CL et al. Preoperative assessment of ureteropelvic junction obstruction with endoluminal sonography and helical CT. AJR Am J Roentgenol 1997; 168: 623–626

Tan BJ, Smith AD. Ureteropelvic junction obstruction repair: when, how, what? Curr Opin Urol 2004; 14: 55–59

Definition

The backward flow of urine from the bladder into the upper urinary tract (ureter, pelvis, and calices).

- **Etiology**
  Developmental abnormality of the UVJ • Incompetence of the one-way valve mechanism at the distal end of the ureter • Often bilateral • Secondary to double ureter or ureteral valves and other anomalies • VUR is graded on a scale of I–V.

Imaging Signs

- **Modality of choice**
  VCUG.
- **Pathognomonic findings**
  Passage of contrast medium from the bladder into the dilated ureter.
- **Voiding cystourethrography findings**
  Retrograde opacification of the (dilated) ureter and also the pelvis and calices with higher-grade reflux • Maximum reflux typically during voiding.
- **Ultrasound and MRI findings**
  Same findings as with VCUG but better evaluation of the renal parenchyma • Both modalities require filling of the bladder with contrast medium (echo enhancer/gadolinium-based agent) • Parenchymal thinning may be present in higher-grade reflux • Limited evaluation of the urethra with both modalities.

Clinical Aspects

- **Typical presentation**
  Recurrent upper UTI.
- **Treatment options**
  Treatment aims to preserve kidney function • Primarily antibiotic prophylaxis • Surgical repair.
- **Course and prognosis**
  Depend on the severity of renal damage at presentation and complications such as reflux nephropathy or chronic pyelonephritis.
- **What does the clinician want to know?**
  Time of occurrence of reflux—already during bladder filling or during voiding • Concomitant anomalies.

Differential Diagnosis

Urinary obstruction	– Antegrade and delayed opacification of the ureter – Mechanical cause (e.g., calculus) visible in most cases

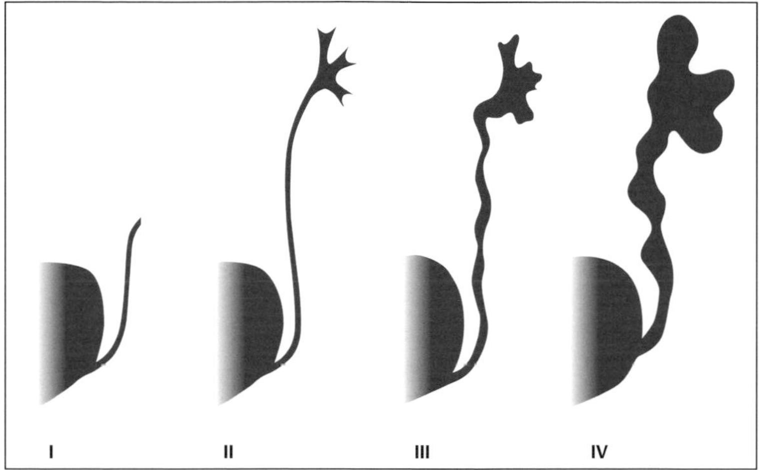

Fig. 2.6 Grading of VUR. Grade I: reflux confined to the lower ureter, which is nondilated; grade II: reflux extends into the ureter, renal pelvis and calices without dilatation; grade III: mild ureteral, pelvic, and caliceal dilatation; grade IV: gross ureteral dilatation and hydronephrosis without elongation of the ureter; grade V: see **Fig. 2.7**.

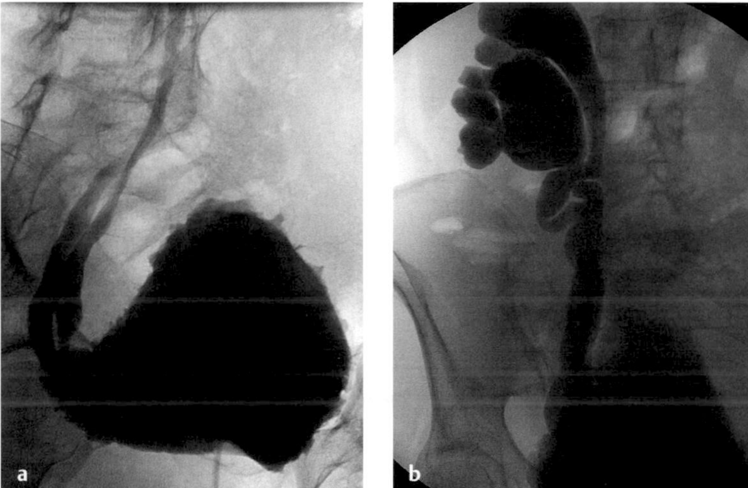

Fig. 2.7 a,b Grade V VUR in a patient with double ureter on the right. VCUG.

a Oblique view of the urinary bladder. Retrograde opacification of both ureters already during filling of the bladder.

b Right kidney. Ballooning of the pelvicaliceal systems and elongation of the ureters.

Tips and Pitfalls

If no postvoid film of the kidneys is obtained, an occasional (usually mild) reflux may be missed because it is suggested only indirectly by retained contrast in the pelvicaliceal system.

Selected References

Berrocal T et al. Anomalies of the distal ureter, bladder, and urethra in children: embryologic, radiologic and pathologic features. Radiographics 2002; 22: 1139–1164

Darge K, Riedmiller H. Current status of vesicoureteral reflux diagnosis. World J Urol 2004; 22: 88–95

Kopac M et al. Indirect voiding urosonography for detecting vesicoureteral reflux in children. Pediatr Nephrol 2005; 20: 1285–1287

Lee SK et al. Magnetic resonance voiding cystography in the diagnosis of vesicoureteral reflux: comparative study with voiding cystoureterography. J Magn Reson Imaging 2005; 21: 406–414

Definition

Any acute blockage of urine flow • Depending on the level of obstruction, the condition affects only a single group of calices (hydrocalix), the entire pelvicaliceal system (hydronephrosis), or the collecting system and ureter (hydroureter).

- **Etiology**
  Mechanical cause (calculus, tumor) in most cases • Obstruction of the urinary tract leads to an increase in intraluminal pressure with subsequent dilatation of the collecting system • *Complication:* Forniceal rupture.

Imaging Signs

- **Modality of choice**
  Ultrasound.
- **Pathognomonic findings**
  Distention of the pelvis and calices without parenchymal atrophy • Prolonged nephrogram.
- **Ultrasound findings**
  Splayed renal pelvis • Dilated anechoic caliceal cups and necks • Kidney may be swollen.
- **CT findings**
  Dilated pelvicaliceal system and possible dilatation of the ureter (0–15 HU) • Delayed renal opacification with delayed excretion • Puddling of contrast medium in the collecting system • Striated perirenal fluid collections.
- **Intravenous pyelogram findings**
  Reduced opacification of the kidney and prolonged nephrogram • Caliceal blunting, splaying, or ballooning, depending on severity • Downward distention of the renal pelvis • Delayed opacification and dilatation of the ureter.

Clinical Aspects

- **Typical presentation**
  Colicky flank pain • Hematuria.
- **Treatment options**
  Elimination of the obstruction (e.g., extraction of a calculus).
- **Course and prognosis**
  Good if promptly diagnosed and treated • *Complications:* Pyelonephritis, forniceal rupture.
- **What does the clinician want to know?**
  Site and cause of the obstruction.

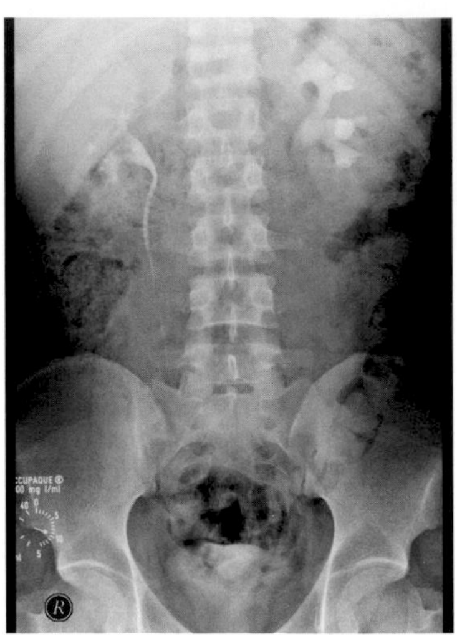

Fig. 2.8 Acute urinary obstruction on the left. IVP 10 minutes after contrast administration. The calices are splayed and opacification of the pelvicaliceal system is less pronounced than on the contralateral side. The left ureter is not yet opacified.

Differential Diagnosis

Chronic urinary obstruction	– Renal parenchymal thinning – Small kidney
Ampullary/extrarenal pelvis	– Normal width of calices and ureter – Nondelayed and symmetric excretion of contrast medium
Parapelvic renal cysts	– No contrast enhancement

Tips and Pitfalls

Small intramural calculi obstructing the ureter are not seen on projection radiographs • CT is indicated in all cases where other modalities fail to identify the cause of acute urinary obstruction.

Selected References

Becker A, Baum M. Obstructive uropathy. Early Hum Dev 2006; 82: 15–22

Dyer RB et al. Classic signs in uroradiology. Radiographics 2004; 24: S247–280

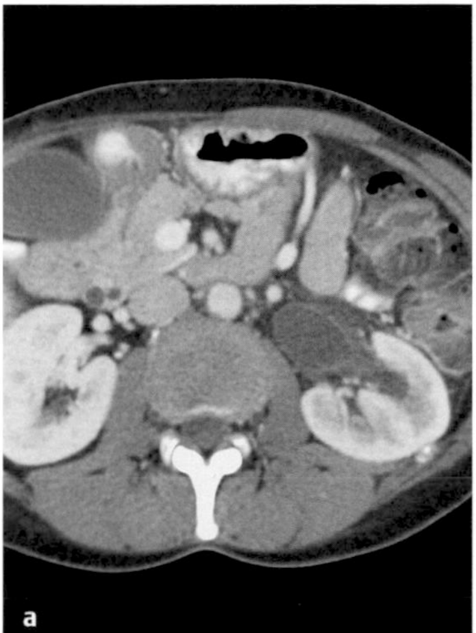

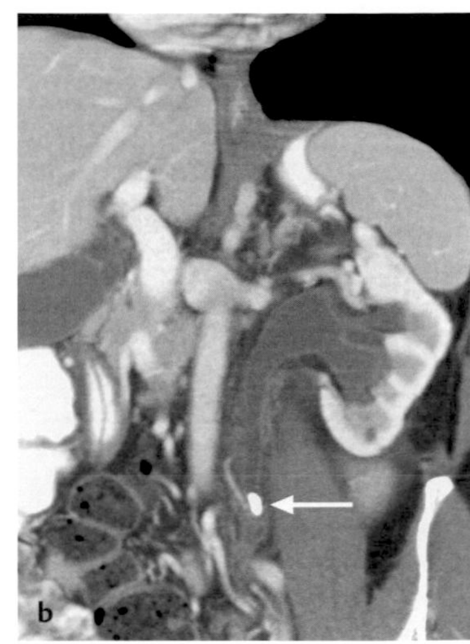

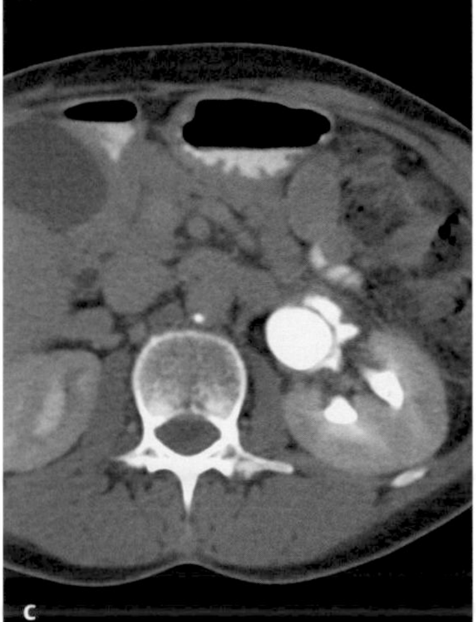

Fig. 2.9 a–c Forniceal rupture secondary to ureteral obstruction by a calculus.

- **a** Corticomedullary phase CT image depicting low-attenuating fluid around the renal pelvis.
- **b** Coronal reconstruction showing a calculus in the upper third of the ureter (arrow) and dilatation of the collecting system.
- **c** Urographic phase CT image showing persistent nephrogram. In addition, enhancement of the peripelvic fluid indicates that the fluid is extravasated urine.

Definition

Prolonged blockage of the urinary tract with renal parenchymal atrophy and loss of renal function, ultimately leading to complete renal failure.

- **Etiology**
  Chronically increased intraluminal pressure • Irreversible pressure atrophy of renal parenchyma • *Causes:* Mechanical (e.g., inflammation) or functional (VUR, neurogenic bladder) • Urinary obstruction leads to muscular hypertrophy of the ureter, which becomes elongated over time • *End stage:* Hydronephrotic kidney.

Imaging Signs

- **Modality of choice**
  CT • MRI in patients with renal dysfunction.
- **Pathognomonic findings**
  Renal parenchymal atrophy • Dilated pelvicaliceal system • Elongated ureter.
- **CT and MRI findings**
  Delayed opacification and excretion • Dilatation of the collecting system and possibly the ureter • Parenchymal thinning • Reduced corticomedullary differentiation.
- **Intravenous pyelogram findings**
  Small kidney with delayed and reduced opacification • Dilatation of the pelvicaliceal system • Tortuous course of the ureter.
- **Ultrasound findings**
  Parenchymal thinning • Caliceal obstruction and dilated pelvicaliceal system.

Clinical Aspects

- **Typical presentation**
  Dull flank pain • Symptoms of the underlying disease (e.g., tumor cachexia) • Pyuria in patients with superinfection.
- **Treatment options**
  Elimination of the underlying pathology • Pressure atrophy of the renal parenchyma is irreversible.
- **Course and prognosis**
  Depend on the extent of renal damage • Urinary obstruction promotes calculus formation and infections (pyelonephritis).
- **What does the clinician want to know?**
  Cause and, if possible, site of the obstruction • Extent of renal parenchymal atrophy.

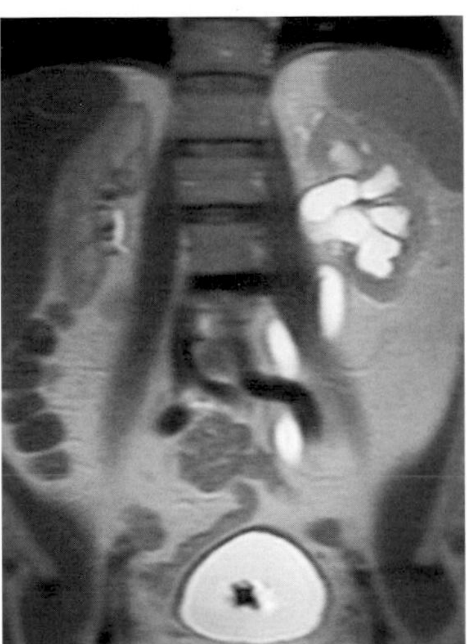

Fig. 2.10 Chronic urinary obstruction on the left in a patient with VUR. Coronal T2-weighted single-shot TSE MR image. There is dilatation of the collecting system and of the elongated ureter. Renal parenchymal thinning. Normal appearance of the right kidney.

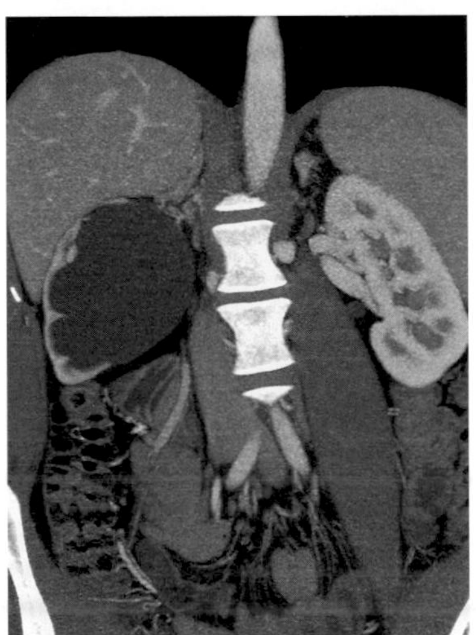

Fig. 2.11 Hydronephrotic kidney on the right, secondary to UPJ stenosis. CT scan showing massive dilatation of the right collecting system and renal atrophy with only a thin margin of residual parenchyma (< 3 mm).

Differential Diagnosis

Acute urinary obstruction	– No renal parenchymal atrophy – Normal-sized or enlarged kidney
Chronic pyelonephritis	– Usually no distention of the collecting system – Cortical depressions

Tips and Pitfalls

Imaging signs of superinfection may be very discreet and are often underestimated • Chronic urinary obstruction is a frequent cause of recurrent UTI.

Selected References

Becker A, Baum M. Obstructive uropathy. Early Hum Dev 2006; 82: 15–22
Dyer RB et al. Classic signs in uroradiology. Radiographics 2004; 24: S247–280

Definition

Proliferation of fibrous and/or chronic inflammatory tissue in the retroperitoneum. *Synonyms:* Idiopathic retroperitoneal fibrosis and Ormond disease.

- **Epidemiology**
  Incidence: 1:200 000 • Three times more common in men • *Peak incidence:* 50–60 years.
- **Etiology**
  Association with periaortitis is assumed • Secondary retroperitoneal fibrosis due to nonspecific inflammation (e.g., following radiotherapy), malignant tumor invasion (breast, colon, stomach, prostate, or uterine cervix), hemorrhage, or certain drugs • Encasement of retroperitoneal structures (ureters, nerves, vessels).

Imaging Signs

- **Modality of choice**
  MRI • Ultrasound for follow-up.
- **Pathognomonic findings**
  Proliferation of fibrous tissue in the retroperitoneal space • Fibrotic process surrounding the aorta and ureters • Medial deviation of the mid-ureters • Concentric ureteral narrowing.
- **MRI findings**
  Retroperitoneal proliferation of fibrous tissue that may extend from the pelvic wall to the renal hilum • Low signal intensity on T1-weighted images • Moderately low signal intensity on T2-weighted images • Encasement of the aorta and ureters • Acute inflammatory episode is indicated by increased signal intensity on T2-weighted images and more marked enhancement • Medial deviation of the ureters • Possible urinary obstruction • Thickening and irregularity of the aortic wall in idiopathic retroperitoneal fibrosis • A highly inhomogeneous appearance on T2-weighted images suggests the malignant form of retroperitoneal fibrosis.
- **Ultrasound findings**
  Hypoechoic deposits of fibrous tissue in the retroperitoneal space • Possible urinary obstruction.
- **CT findings**
  Low-attenuating fibrous tissue in the retroperitoneum • Otherwise same as on MRI.
- **Intravenous pyelogram findings**
  Medial deviation of the mid-ureters • Extrinsic (concentric) ureteral compression • Possible pelvicaliceal dilatation.

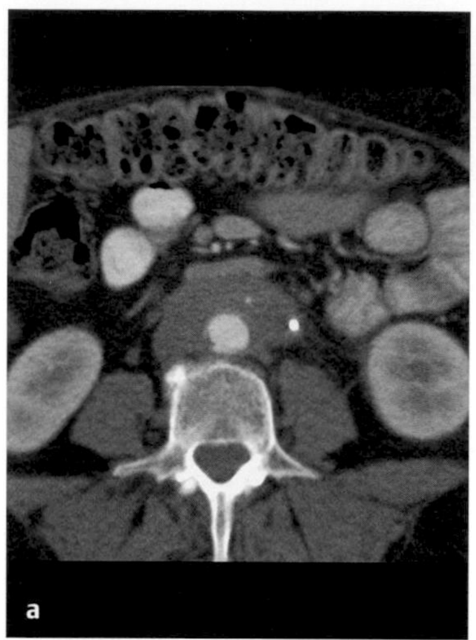

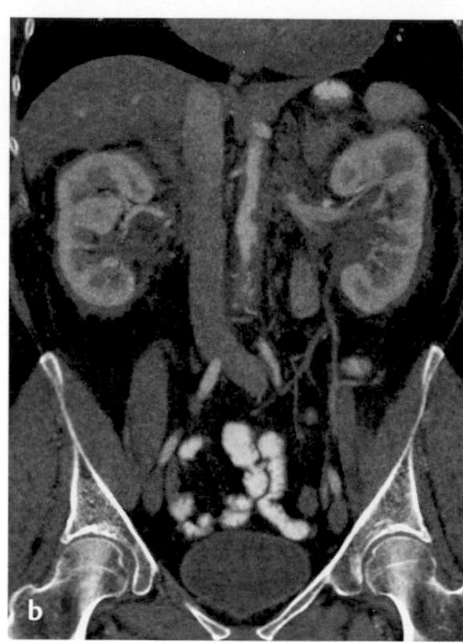

Fig. 2.12 a, b Retroperitoneal fibrosis. CT.

a Hypodense fibrous tissue surrounding the aorta, inferior mesenteric artery, and left ureter (ureteral stent).

b Coronal reconstruction showing the extent of the fibrotic process and involvement of both kidneys. In addition, there are wall irregularities of the aorta.

Clinical Aspects

- **Typical presentation**
  Symptoms are nonspecific • Diffuse, dull back pain • Weight loss • Leg lymphedema.
- **Treatment options**
  No curative treatment for idiopathic retroperitoneal fibrosis; primary aim is to preserve renal function • Steroids and/or immunosuppression • Ureteral stenting • Nephrostomy • If possible, elimination of the cause in secondary retroperitoneal fibrosis.
- **Course and prognosis**
  Insidious course • Good prognosis if renal function is preserved.
- **What does the clinician want to know?**
  Organs involved • Presence of hydronephrosis • Extent of inflammatory process.

Differential Diagnosis

Urothelial carcinoma of the ureter	– Circumscribed eccentric ureteral stenosis – Ureteral dilatation proximal and distal to the tumor
Retroperitoneal lymphadenopathy	– Enlarged lymph nodes, typically with lateral ureteral displacement – Tends to be more proximal (upper third of ureter and above) – Anterior displacement of the aorta and vena cava

Selected References

Vaglio A et al. Retroperitoneal fibrosis. Lancet 2006; 367: 241–251

Vivas I et al. Retroperitoneal fibrosis: typical and atypical manifestations. Br J Radiol 2000; 73: 214–222

Definition

The presence of calculi in the renal collecting system (nephrolithiasis), ureter (ureterolithiasis), or urinary bladder (urocystolithiasis) • Less common are calculi in the renal papillae (parenchymal calculi) • Minute calculi are also referred to as *gravel*.

- **Epidemiology**
  More common in men than women • *Peak incidence:* Fifth decade.
- **Etiology and pathophysiology**
  The following types (percentage, causes) are distinguished according to composition:
  - Calcium oxalate (60%, hyperoxaluria, primary hyperparathyroidism, idiopathic hypercalciuria)—opaque.
  - Calcium phosphate (20%, renal tubular acidosis)—opaque.
  - Uric acid (5–15%, hyperuricemia)—nonopaque.
  - Cystine (1%, cystinuria)—very faintly opaque.
  - Struvite (10–20%, infection with urease-producing bacteria)—faintly opaque.

  Lithogenic factors: Increased urine excretion (calcium, oxalate, uric acid) • Lack of inhibitors (citrate, pyrophosphate) • Abnormal urinary pH (low pH: uric acid calculi; high pH: struvite calculi) • Recurrent UTI.

Imaging Signs

- **Modality of choice**
  Ultra-low-dose CT (unenhanced), plain abdominal film (supine KUB).
- **CT findings**
  Rounded high-attenuating intraluminal structure • CT allows precise definition of calculus location, especially in relation to the ureter.
- **Radiographic findings**
  Rounded density projected over the renal collecting system or the ureter • An occasional calculus may conform to the contour of a calix (staghorn calculus) • *Location:* Any of the three major caliceal groups, caliceal neck, renal pelvis, ureter, ureterovesical junction (prevesical) • A radiolucent calculus is seen only indirectly as a filling defect after contrast administration.
- **Intravenous pyelogram findings**
  Exact location relative to the caliceal group, caliceal neck, renal pelvis, or ureter • Radiolucent calculi are seen as smooth filling defects • Ureteral dilatation that ends abruptly as an indirect sign of a calculus causing urinary obstruction (hydroureter, hydronephrosis).
- **Ultrasound findings**
  Highly echogenic focus with acoustic shadowing (which may be absent when the calculus is small) • Ureteral calculi are difficult to detect by ultrasound.

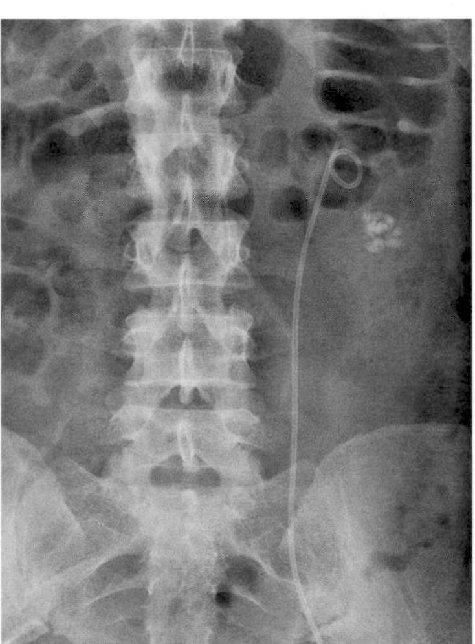

Fig. 2.13 Urolithiasis. KUB. Multiple clustered calculi in the lower group of calices of the left kidney (a double-J stent lies in the ureter).

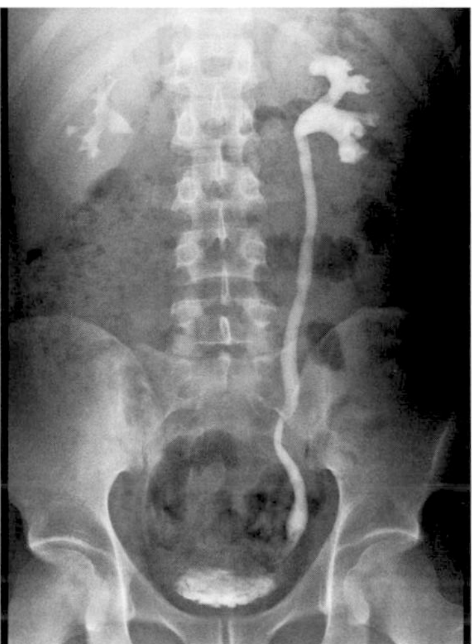

Fig. 2.14 Calculus in the distal third of the left ureter. Postvoid radiograph after intravenous contrast administration. The dilated ureter tapers toward the obstructing calculus.

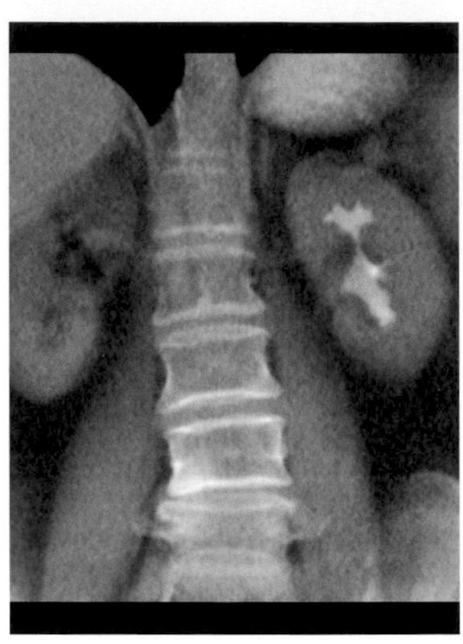

Fig. 2.15 Staghorn calculus in the left pelvicaliceal system. Coronal CT reconstruction from unenhanced ultra-low-dose CT data.

Clinical Aspects

- **Typical presentation**
  Colicky flank pain • Often associated with nausea and vomiting • Hematuria.
- **Treatment options**
  Depend on location, size, and clinical symptoms • *Nonsurgical management:* Shock wave lithotripsy (ESWL) • *Surgical:* Ureteroscopic or percutaneous approach; laparoscopic anatrophic nephrolithotomy may be required to remove a staghorn calculus • Small asymptomatic caliceal stones do not necessarily require treatment.
- **Course and prognosis**
  Patients with nephrolithiasis have a 10-year recurrence rate of 50% and a 20-year recurrence rate of 75% • The underlying predisposing condition is usually not identified.
- **What does the clinician want to know?**
  Number, size, and location of calculi (e.g., caliceal neck) • Follow-up after intervention (e.g., multiple small stone particles in the ureter ("steinstrasse") after lithotripsy).

Differential Diagnosis

Phlebolith	– Smooth rounded mass – Central lucency
Calcified mesenteric lymph node	– Morphology (lobulated, plaquelike) – May change position (mesentery)
Nephrocalcinosis	– Stippled calcifications, mainly involving the pyramids – May be confined to a wedge-shaped area
Vascular calcifications	– Linear
Coproliths	– May occur anywhere in the colon (typically in the appendix) – Central lucency – Inhomogeneous

Tips and Pitfalls

A calculus obscured by an overlying transverse process may be missed • Projection radiography is limited in the presence of coprostasis.

Selected References

Deger S et al. Laparoscopic anatrophic nephrolithotomy. Scand J Urol Nephrol 2004; 38: 263–265

Moe OW. Kidney stones: pathophysiology and medical management. Lancet 2006; 376: 333–344

Sandhu C. Urinary tract stones—Part I: role of radiological imaging in diagnosis and treatment planning. Clin Radiol 2003; 58: 415–421

Straub M et al. Diagnosis and metaphylaxis of stone disease. World J Urol 2005; 23: 309–323

Definition

- **Etiology**
  Iatrogenic trauma (pelvic surgery) • Penetrating trauma (gunshot or stab wound) • Blunt trauma sustained in deceleration accidents (rare, typically involving the UPJ) • Severity ranges from partial tear to ureteral avulsion • Intraperitoneal or retroperitoneal injury.

Imaging Signs

- **Modality of choice**
  CT with urographic/delayed phase.
- **Pathognomonic findings**
  Extravasation of contrast medium • Urinary ascites.
- **CT findings**
  Extravasated contrast medium • Urinary ascites • Reduced or absent opacification of the ureter below the level of injury • Retroperitoneal urinoma may be present • Obstructive changes ranging from dilatation of the proximal urinary tract to acute hydronephrosis.
- **Intravenous pyelogram findings**
  Soft tissue shadow projected over the ureter (urinoma) • Extravasation of contrast medium • Displacement of the ureter and possibly also the kidney • Prolonged nephrogram.

Clinical Aspects

- **Typical presentation**
  Flank pain • Hematuria • Ascites (urinary).
- **Treatment options**
  Initial conservative management in patients without dehiscence (nephrostomy and antibiotic therapy) • Suture repair in case of dehiscence • Possible retrograde pyelogram and stent placement.
- **Course and prognosis**
  Good prognosis in most cases • Ureteral anastomosis is technically very demanding • Most frequent complication: urinoma.
- **What does the clinician want to know?**
  Concomitant injuries.

Differential Diagnosis

Urothelial carcinoma	– Filling defect – No contrast extravasation – Dilatation of the ureteral segments proximal and distal to the tumor

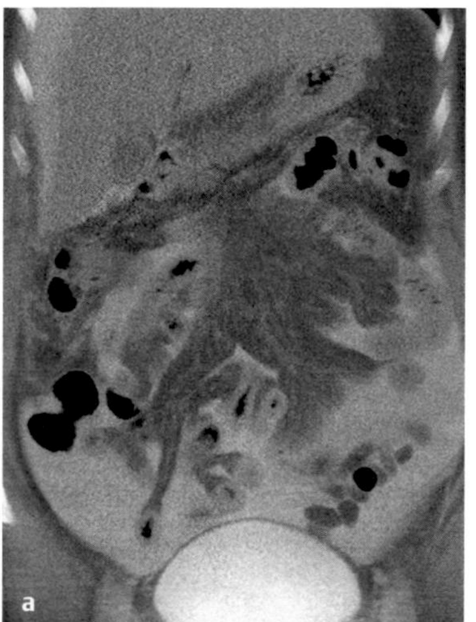

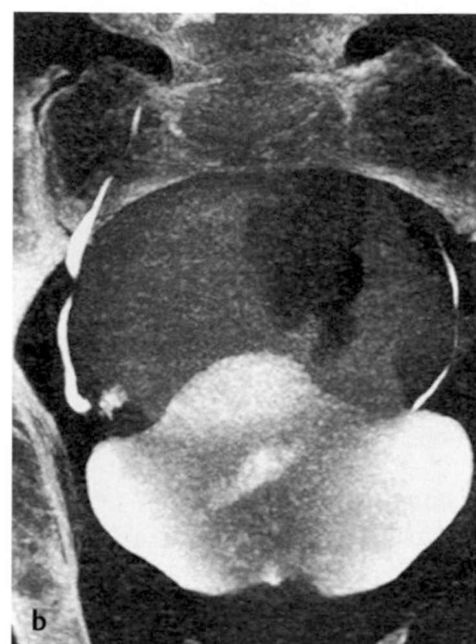

Fig. 2.16 a, b Injury to the right ureter in the true pelvis.

a Ultra-low-dose CT scan obtained 30 minutes after contrast administration. High-attenuating ascites around the liver and in the middle and lower abdomen.

b CT urography (coronal MIP reconstruction). The extravasated contrast medium indicates the exact site of perforation of the lower ureter.

Tips and Pitfalls

Ureteral injury must be considered in the differential diagnosis in patients with postoperative ascites • Hematuria may be absent if there is complete avulsion of the ureter.

Selected References

Goldman SM, Sandler CM. Urogenital trauma: imaging upper GU trauma. Eur J Radiol 2004; 50: 84–95

Titton R et al. Urine leaks and urinomas: diagnosis and imaging-guided intervention. Radiographics 2003; 23: 1133–1147

Wah TM, Spencer JA. The role of CT in the management of adult urinary tract trauma. Clin Radiol 2001; 56: 268–277

Definition

Carcinoma arising in the epithelium of the upper urinary tract.

- **Epidemiology**
  Three times more common in men than women • *Peak incidence:* Sixth decade • Annual incidence in Europe and the USA: 20 in 100 000.
- **Etiology**
  Smoking is the single most important risk factor • A genetic disposition has been proposed but its influence seems to be small • Papillary carcinoma is the most common type • Muscle invasion (T2 tumors) is paramount for staging, treatment, and prognosis.

Imaging Signs

- **Modality of choice**
  Biphasic CT with CT IVP.
- **Pathognomonic findings**
  Irregular polypoid filling defect in the collecting system.
- **CT and MRI findings**
  Irregular polypoid intraluminal mass with only slight contrast enhancement • The collecting system proximal and distal to the tumor may be enlarged.
- **Intravenous pyelogram findings**
  Isolated or multiple filling defects within the collecting system • Dilatation of a single calix (hydrocalix) or the entire collecting system (hydronephrosis, hydroureter).

Clinical Aspects

- **Typical presentation**
  Painless hematuria.
- **Treatment options**
  Curative: Radical resection (nephroureterectomy with partial bladder resection) • *Palliative:* Radiotherapy, chemotherapy.
- **Course and prognosis**
  Depend on the T stage • Well-differentiated in situ and T1 tumors have a very good prognosis • Patients with muscle infiltration (T2) have a much poorer prognosis • T3/T4 tumors have a 5-year survival rate of less than 20%.
- **What does the clinician want to know?**
  Extent: Panurothelial disease • Severity of urinary obstruction • Tumor stage.

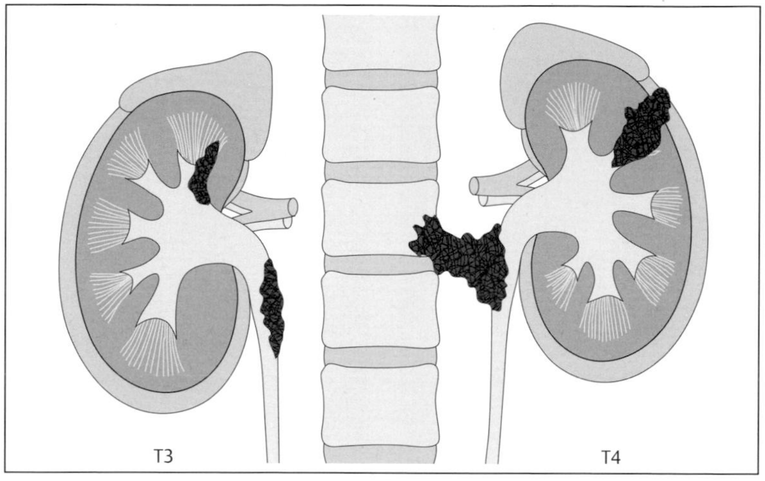

Fig. 2.17 T3/T4 stages of urothelial carcinoma of the renal pelvis and ureter. T3 tumors extend beyond the muscularis propria and invade the peripelvic/periureteral tissue or renal parenchyma. T4 tumors invade perirenal fat or contiguous organs.

Differential Diagnosis

Renal cell carcinoma	– Hypervascular tumor – Predominantly intraparenchymal – Tumor may extend into the renal vein – No urinary obstruction
Renal tuberculosis	– Bizarre morphology – Calcifications
Radiolucent calculus	– Smooth contour – No contrast enhancement – Ureteral spasm distal to the calculus

Tips and Pitfalls

Panurothelial disease: Imaging must include the lower urinary tract and contralateral collecting system in order not to underestimate tumor extent • A tumor may be missed on IVP unless at least three zonograms are obtained.

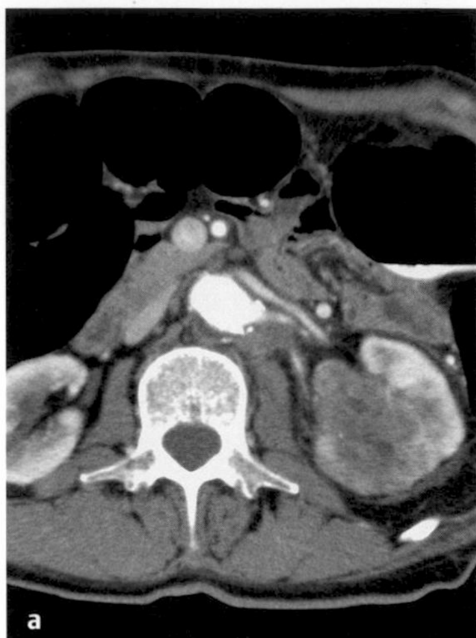

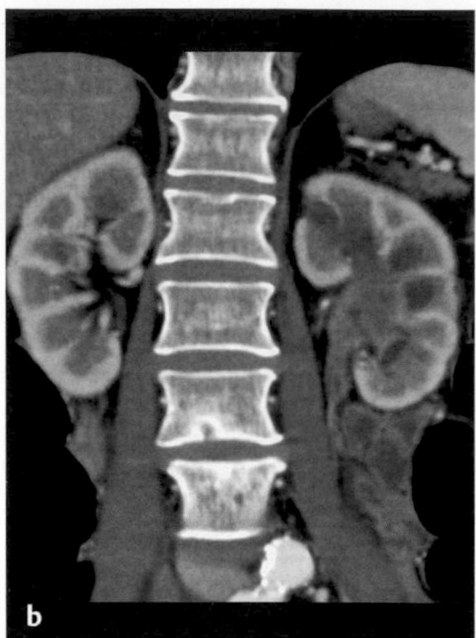

Fig. 2.18 a, b Urothelial carcinoma (T4) of the left kidney extending from the renal pelvis into the proximal ureter.

a Axial corticomedullary phase CT scan. Inhomogeneous opacification of the tumor, which is seen to extend through the posterior parenchyma into the perinephric fatty tissue.

b Coronal reconstruction showing dilated calices and extension of the tumor into the proximal ureter.

Selected References

Browne RF et al. Transitional cell carcinoma of the upper urinary tract: spectrum of imaging findings. Radiographics 2005; 25: 1609–1627

Caoili EM et. al. MDCT urography of upper tract urothelial neoplasms. AJR Am J Roentgenol 2005; 184: 1873–1881

Definition

Pouches of the urinary bladder involving all layers of the wall • The condition is known as *pseudodiverticulum* if only the mucosa protrudes through a weak spot in the detrusor muscle of the bladder • Bladder tumors may arise in a diverticulum (increased risk of intradiverticular development of urothelial cancer due to retention of carcinogenic substances in the pouch).

- **Epidemiology**
  Acquired bladder diverticula develop secondary to bladder outlet obstruction (benign prostatic hyperplasia, prostate cancer, urethral stricture), therefore their incidence increases with age, and they are rare in women.
- **Etiology**
  Typically due to increased intravesical pressure as a result of bladder outlet obstruction.

Imaging Signs

- **Modality of choice**
  Conventional radiography, ultrasound.
- **Projection radiographic findings**
  Bladder diverticula can be diagnosed using IVP, cystography, or VCUG • Depending on their location, diverticula may opacify later than the normal bladder lumen • Radiographs should be obtained in several planes and under fluoroscopy to ensure visualization of the entire bladder circumference • Evaluation comprises site, shape, and contour of the diverticula • A diverticulum with a narrow neck may show persistent opacification after voiding.
- **Ultrasound findings**
  Adequate evaluation possible only with the bladder filled to at least 200 mL • Pouches in the bladder wall • Anechoic urine in the diverticulum.
- **CT and MRI**
  Multiphasic CT and MRI (during the corticomedullary phase, e.g., 60 seconds after the start of contrast administration, and additional late images 10–15 minutes after the end of contrast administration) • Thin-slice reconstruction and, depending on the shape of the diverticulum, multiplanar reconstruction or angulated plane in MRI.

Clinical Aspects

- **Typical presentation**
  Patients with acquired bladder diverticula typically present with symptoms of the underlying disease that causes bladder outlet obstruction.
- **Treatment options**
  Surgical removal may be considered in patients with large diverticula.
- **Course and prognosis**
  Retention of urine in a diverticulum promotes tumor development • Recurrent UTI.

Fig. 2.19 Bladder diverticula. VCUG. There is good visualization of the bladder diverticula using rotating fluoroscopy.

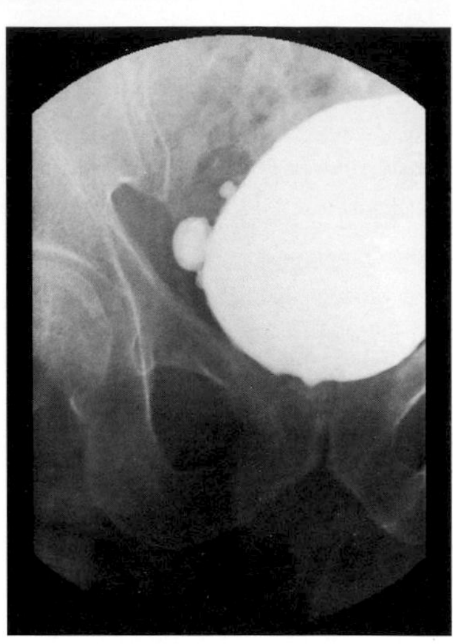

▸ **What does the clinician want to know?**
Site • Size • Complications (signs of inflammation, tumor).

Differential Diagnosis

Paravesical cysts, e.g., ovarian cysts	– Topographic relationship to uterine appendages – No neck
Urachal cyst	– Cystic or ductlike structure located in the midline anterior to the bladder and extending to the umbilicus
Bladder perforation	– Contrast leakage into surrounding tissue – No enclosing structure such as a wall – Irregular contour (history of trauma or operation?)
Bladder tumor with extravesical extension	– No fluid-filled center – Changes in the bladder wall

Tips and Pitfalls

Perform projection radiography in more than one plane • Obtain late images when performing contrast-enhanced MRI or CT • Ensure adequate bladder filling.

Selected References

Beyersdorff D. Harnblase. In: Freyschmidt, Nicolas, Heywang-Köbrunner (eds). Handbuch für Radiologie. Heidelberg: Springer; 2004

Dunnick NR et al (eds). Textbook of Uroradiology. The Urinary Bladder/Diverticula. Philadelphia: Lippincott Williams & Wilkins; 2001: 362–364

Definition

- **Epidemiology**
  Most frequent malignant tumor of the urinary bladder • 93% of urinary tract neoplasms are found in the bladder and 3% each in the pelvicaliceal system and ureters • Polypoid growth is the most common form • Incidence increases with age • Estimated incidence of bladder cancer in the USA in 2006: 61420 cases • *Risk factors:* Smoking, environmental toxins.
- **Staging of bladder carcinoma**
  Stage TA: Superficial tumor.
  Stage T1: Infiltration of submucosa.
  Stage T2a: Infiltration of superficial muscle.
  Stage T2b: Infiltration of deep muscle.
  Stage T3: Extension to perivesical fat.
  Stage T4: Extension to adjacent organs (prostate, uterus, rectum, pelvic floor muscles).
  Stage N1: A minimal axial diameter over 10 mm is suggestive of lymph node metastasis.

Imaging Signs

- **Modality of choice**
  Routine workup:
  - Initial cystoscopy with TURB.
  - IVP with tomogram of the pelvicaliceal system; alternatively multislice CT with an additional late scan 10 minutes after the start of contrast administration (CTU).
  - Abdominal CT (lymph node evaluation).
  - Chest radiograph.

  MRI of the true pelvis will show the depth of infiltration and, where present, extension to adjacent organs. MRI is superior only if CT is performed on a single-row scanner or no thin-slice reconstruction of the CT data set is available.
- **Intravenous pyelogram findings**
  Plain film • Intravenous administration of 100 mL nonionic contrast medium containing 300 mg iodine/g • Abdominal films 10 and 20 minutes post contrast • At least two tomograms between 10 and 20 minutes after contrast administration • Postvoid film with the patient standing (and with the catheter clamped off in patients with an indwelling bladder catheter) • Carefully look for urinary obstruction or filling defects that indicate tumor location or a second tumor site.

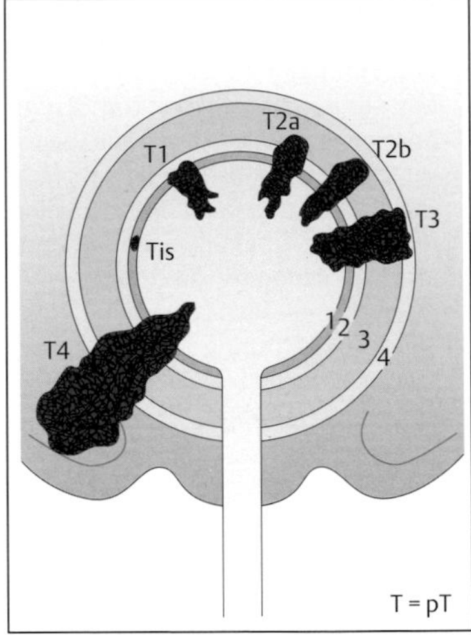

Fig. 2.20 Stages of urothelial carcinoma of the bladder.
1 Epithelium
2 Subepithelial connective tissue
3 Muscle
4 Perivesical fat

- **CT findings**
  Bladder should be at least moderately filled • Multiphasic scan with thin-slice reconstruction • First phase 50 seconds after intravenous administration of 120 mL of a nonionic iodine-based contrast medium • Second phase 10 minutes post contrast when opacification of the pelvicaliceal system, ureters, and bladder has occurred • A polypoid mass or wall thickening is indicative of urothelial carcinoma • Multiplanar reconstruction where required.
- **MRI findings**
  Bladder should be at least moderately filled • Axial and coronal T2-weighted TSE sequences and axial T1-weighted sequences • Slice thickness: 4 mm • T2-weighted sequence perpendicular to the tumor base where needed • Additional axial PD-weighted sequence covering the area up to the aortic bifurcation (lymph nodes) • Dynamic T1-weighted sequence perpendicular to the tumor base before and 15, 55, 120, and 300 seconds after intravenous administration of gadolinium DTPA • Bladder tumors typically enhance early, which is why in most cases the depth of bladder wall invasion can be determined on early post-contrast images.

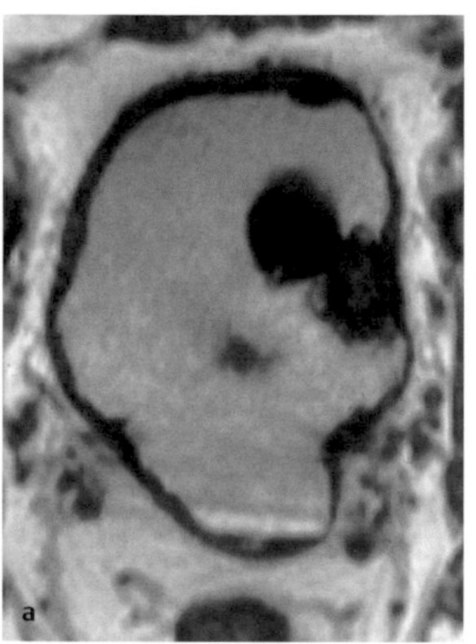

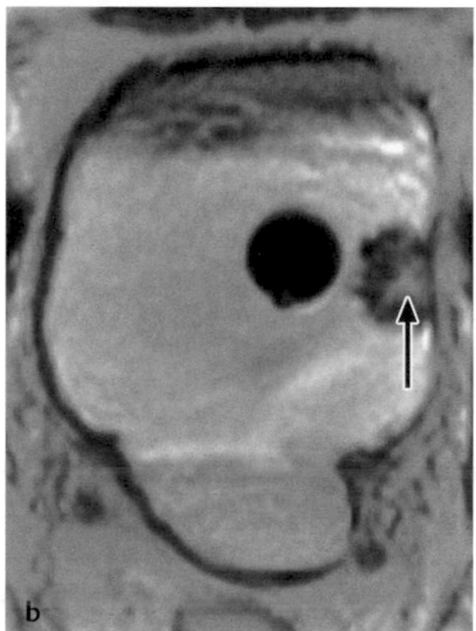

Fig. 2.21 a, b Axial T1-weighted MRI.

a Polypoid mass arising from the left wall (balloon catheter adjacent to the tumor). High signal intensity of the bladder contents due to contrast medium.

b Good visualization of the bladder wall and the polypoid mass (arrow). There is central enhancement of the tumor following intravenous administration of a nonspecific gadolinium-based contrast medium.

Clinical Aspects

- **Typical presentation**
  Microscopic hematuria • Gross hematuria • Urinary retention and obstruction are late sequelae • Thrombosis in case of tumor extension to the pelvic wall • Deteriorating general condition in patients with metastatic disease.
- **Treatment options**
  Transurethral resection of superficial tumor • Radical cystectomy with creation of a neobladder for tumors invading the submucosa and muscle • Ileal conduit after cystectomy for higher-stage tumors.
- **Course and prognosis**
  Patients with superficial bladder cancer have a 5-year survival rate of 90% • Bladder cancer invading the pelvic wall can cause pelvic thrombosis • Lymphatic and hematogenous metastatic spread to the liver, lungs, and bones in advanced bladder cancer.
- **What does the clinician want to know?**
  Location of the tumor • Depth of bladder wall invasion • Tumor extent beyond the bladder • Lymph node enlargement • Additional suspicious filling defects in the pelvicaliceal system and ureters.

Differential Diagnosis

Rectum/uterus	– Typical impressions of the superior and posterior aspects of the bladder
Crossing vessels	– Identified as such on CT scans and by the orientation of the filling defects on IVP
Scars, granulomas	– Difficult to distinguish in most cases—cystoscopic biopsy
Mucosal folds	– Examination with a filled bladder

Tips and Pitfalls

Perform examinations with the bladder filled to at least 200 mL to ensure adequate distention and optimal evaluation • Clamp off the bladder catheter • Obtain additional late-phase CT scan.

Selected References

Beyersdorff D. Harnblase. In: Freyschmidt J et al (eds). Handbuch für Radiologie. Heidelberg: Springer; 2004

Wong-You-Cheong JJ et al. From the archives of the AFIP: Neoplasms of the urinary bladder: radiologic-pathologic correlation. Radiographics 2006; 26: 553–580

Definition

Narrowing of the bulbar and penile urethra • Physiologic narrowing of the membranous urethra by the urethral sphincter • Congenital stricture due to urethral valve.

- **Etiology**
  After infection, especially gonorrhea • After trauma.

Imaging Signs

- **Modality of choice**
  Retrograde urethrogram.
- **Retrograde urethrogram**
  Typically indicated to exclude stricture of the urethra in patients presenting with reduced urine flow and suspected BPH • Evaluation of the urethra under fluoroscopic control after administration of an iodine-based contrast medium • Air-contrast study in cases of air inclusions or questionable strictures.
- **Ultrasound findings**
  Ultrasound will depict wall changes but does not allow evaluation of urethral stricture.

Clinical Aspects

- **Typical presentation**
  Reduced urine flow during voiding • Voiding may be painful • Recurrence of strictures is common.
- **Treatment options**
  Depend on length of stricture and course • Dilatation • Urethral anastomosis • Mesh graft • Suprapubic drainage in patients with acute urinary retention.
- **Course and prognosis**
  Patients with untreated urethral stricture may develop all complications associated with bladder outlet obstruction: trabeculated bladder, VUR, and urinary obstruction • The recurrence rate varies with the underlying cause and type of stricture.
- **What does the clinician want to know?**
  Location and extent of the stricture.

Differential Diagnosis

BPH	– Reduced urine flow during voiding but no stricture of the penile and bulbar urethra
Urethral rupture	– Contrast leakage during retrograde urethrography
Urethral tumor	– Induration – Solid tumor (rare)

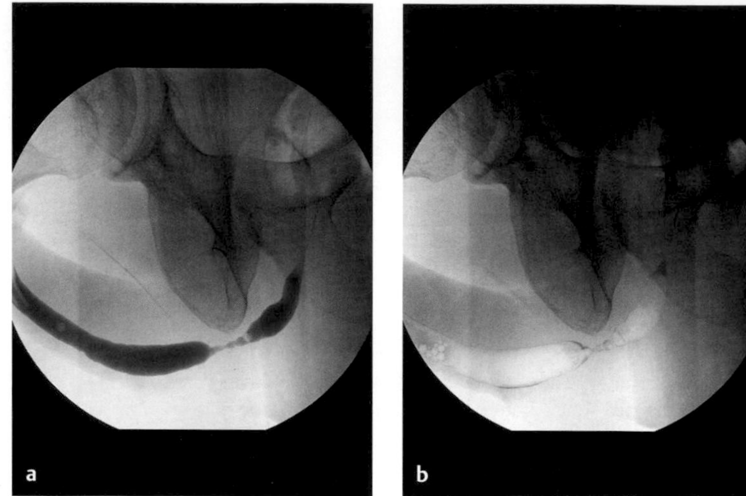

Fig. 2.22 a, b Retrograde urethrogram. Stricture of the bulbar urethra after gonorrhea before (**a**) and after introduction of air (**b**).

Tips and Pitfalls

Optimal evaluation with the penile urethra straightened and the pelvis tilted 40° toward the examiner for evaluation of the bulbar urethra • Flush catheter to remove air before contrast injection.

Selected References

Pavlica P et al. Imaging of male urethra. Review Eur Radiol 2003; 13: 1583–1596

Definition

- *Urethral diverticula:* Most acquired diverticula develop from periurethral glands • Typically open into the posterolateral part of the middle or distal urethra.
- *Urethral tumors:* Very rare • Squamous cell carcinoma is the most common urethral tumor, followed by urothelial carcinoma and adenocarcinoma.
- Fistulas terminating in the urethra.

► **Epidemiology**

1.4% of patients presenting with stress urinary incontinence have urethral diverticula • Urethral tumors are four times more common in women than men.

Imaging Signs

► **Modality of choice**

Routine diagnostic workup:

- Clinical examination: A diverticulum or tumor of the urethra is palpated as a firm mass.
- Double-balloon urethrography (DBU): Serves to search for a fistula terminating in the urethra or an ectopic ureter and to exclude urethral diverticula.
- MRI: May be indicated to evaluate patients with tumors and complex cysts
- Ultrasound: Presence of an anechoic paraurethral lesion does not allow differentiation between a diverticulum and paraurethral cyst.

► **Double-balloon urethrography**

Performed on the fluoroscopy table with the patient supine • The double-balloon catheter is advanced into the bladder to occlude the neck with the proximal balloon • The moveable distal balloon is then pushed against the external urethral meatus • Contrast medium is injected into the catheter and enters the urethra via a side hole • With this technique, not only the urethra but also diverticula and fistulas can be opacified with a minimum of pressure.

► **MRI findings**

Imaging with the body phased-array coil • At least two sequences perpendicular to each other • Urethral anatomy (target appearance) is best appreciated on PD-weighted or T2-weighted images • Slice thickness of 3–4 mm • Paraurethral cysts and diverticula have high signal intensity on T2-weighted images.

► **Ultrasound findings**

Ultrasound is performed with a vaginal sector scanner with at least 5 MHz • Good delineation of the urethra, surrounding tissues, and the urinary bladder • Cysts and fluid-filled diverticula are depicted as smooth lesions without internal echoes • Sediment may be present.

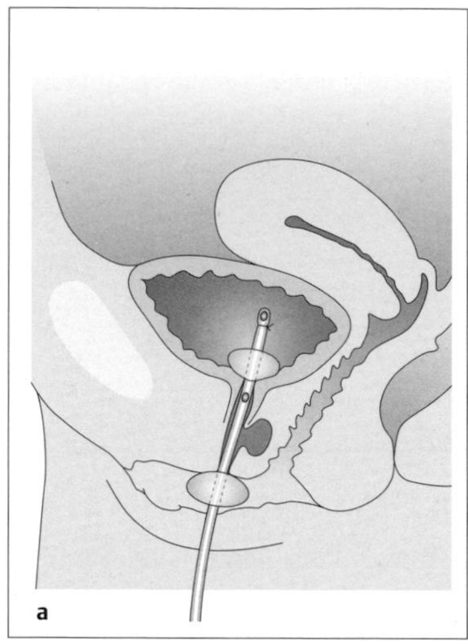

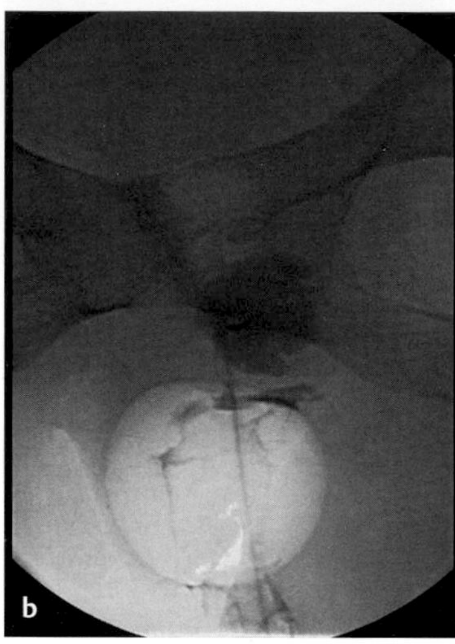

Fig. 2.23 a, b Urethral diverticulum.
a Diagrammatic representation of double-balloon urethrography.
b Opacification of the urethra and diverticulum by contrast medium exiting the catheter via a side hole (oblique view).

Clinical Aspects

- **Typical presentation**
  Urethral diverticula typically present with the "three Ds": dysuria, postvoid dribbling, and dyspareunia.
- **Treatment options**
  Resection of the diverticulum or cyst.
- **Course and prognosis**
  Good prognosis after diverticulum resection • Doubtful prognosis in patients with urethral tumor.
- **What does the clinician want to know?**
  Differentiation of paraurethral cysts and diverticula • Site of the neck if a diverticulum has been demonstrated.

Differential Diagnosis

Urethral tumor	– Firm mass, solid
Paraurethral cyst	– High signal intensity on T2-weighted images – No contrast uptake on double-balloon urethrography
Urethral diverticulum	– High signal intensity on T2-weighted images – Contrast uptake on double-balloon urethrography

Selected References

Golomb J et al. Comparison of voiding cystourethrography and double-balloon urethrography in the diagnosis of complex female urethral diverticula. European Radiology 2003; 13: 536–542

Kawashima A et al. Imaging of urethral disease: A pictorial review. Radiographics 2004; 24: S195–216

Tunn R et al. Diagnostik von Urethradivertikeln und periurethralen Raumforderungen. Fortschr Röntgenstr 2001; 173: 109–114

Definition

The following pelvic fistulas are distinguished according to site: vesicovaginal, rectovaginal, vesicoenteric or vesicorectal, and vesicocutaneous fistulas.

► **Etiology**
Inflammation • Tumor • Surgery • Radiotherapy.

Imaging Signs

► **Modality of choice**
Routine diagnostic workup: To evaluate the course of the fistula tract suspected on the basis of the patient's symptoms:
- Clinical examination.
- Cystoscopy.
- Cystography under fluoroscopy if the course of the tract is not definitely clear.
- May be supplemented by VCUG to identify urethral fistulas and very small fistulas that become patent only through the increased intravesical pressure occurring during voiding.

Ultrasound and MRI have limited roles • MRI precisely outlines the course of a fistula tract through soft tissue.

► **MRI findings**
MRI is performed with the body phased-array coil • Angulated axial and coronal T2-weighted TSE sequences and axial T1-weighted sequences • Slice thickness: 3 mm • Fistulas have high signal intensity on TIRM images • Additional T1-weighted, fat-saturated sequences after intravenous administration of contrast medium • Most urinary fistulas are less conspicuous than anal fistulas because they cause only little reaction in the surrounding tissue.

Clinical Aspects

► **Typical presentation**
Recurrent UTI • Passage of air with the urine • Urine in stool • Signs of inflammation • Pain • Prior surgery or radiotherapy and the duration of symptoms provide important clues.

► **Treatment options**
Complete resection and repair • Catheterization to relieve the bladder • Stoma to relieve the rectum in the presence of rectal fistula.

► **Course and prognosis**
Risk of recurrence varies with the underlying disease • Outcome depends on whether complete repair is achieved.

► **What does the clinician want to know?**
Site of origin and termination of the fistula • Exact course.

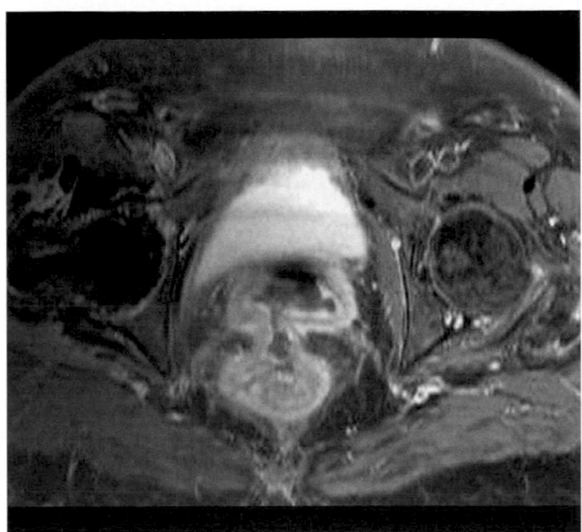

Fig. 2.24 Rectovaginal fistula. Axial T1-weighted MR image after intravenous contrast administration. Large cervical carcinoma with tumor fistula extending from the necrotic cavity to the rectum.

Differential Diagnosis: Causes of Fistula

Tumor	– Tumor infiltrating the bladder: MRI
Inflammation	– History – Inflammatory fistula associated with higher recurrence rate
Surgery/radiotherapy	– History – Cystography, VCUG – MRI may be indicated to exclude recurrent tumor

Selected References

Kavanagh D et al. Diagnosis and treatment of enterovesical fistulae. Colorectal Dis 2005; 7: 286–291

Semelka RC et al. Pelvic fistulas: appearance on MR images. Abdom Imaging 1997; 22: 91–95

Definition

The most common operations on the lower urinary tract are:
- *TURP:* For benign prostatic hyperplasia.
- *TURB:* For diagnosis and treatment of polypoid bladder tumors • Often repeat intervention due to tumor recurrence.
- *Radical prostatectomy:* For prostate cancer without extracapsular extension • Anastomosis of the bladder and urethra.
- *Cystectomy with creation of a neobladder:* For localized tumors of the bladder • Bladder substitute constructed from an ileal segment • Ureteral reimplantation and urethral anastomosis.
- *Urethral surgery:* For urethral rupture, urethral injury associated with penile trauma, long or recurrent strictures • Dilatation, longitudinal incision, end-to-end anastomosis, or mesh graft.

Radiographic follow-up of anastomoses.

Imaging Signs

▸ **Modality of choice**
VCUG, may be supplemented by retrograde urethrogram.
Routine diagnostic workup: VCUG follow-up of anastomoses and sutures after prostatectomy and cystectomy • Administration of an iodine-based contrast medium via a bladder catheter under fluoroscopy until the patient has a desire to void (extravasation?) • Rotating fluoroscopy • Evaluation of voiding.

▸ **Findings**
- *TURP:* Central craterlike defect in the prostate.
- *TURB:* Irregularities and focal lesions of the bladder wall • No routine postoperative radiographic follow-up needed.
- *Radical prostatectomy:* Control of the anastomosis with the postoperative bladder catheter in place • If the anastomosis is intact (no extravasation), evaluation of postoperative urinary continence (start-and-stop test).
- *Cystectomy with creation of a neobladder:* Bladder substitute consisting of an ileal loop with an irregular contour • Exclusion of extravasation and evaluation of voiding.
- *Urethral surgery:* Routine radiologic follow-up not necessary in all cases • Retrograde urethrogram may be indicated • Alternatively, antegrade urethrogram in patients with a suprapubic catheter in place.

▸ **What does the clinician want to know?**
Extravasation • Presence of stenoses • Evaluation of continence after prostatectomy.

Tips and Pitfalls

Contrast administration should always be done under fluoroscopy for timely identification of extravasation • Otherwise site of extravasation may be obscured by too much contrast medium • VCUG in at least two planes.

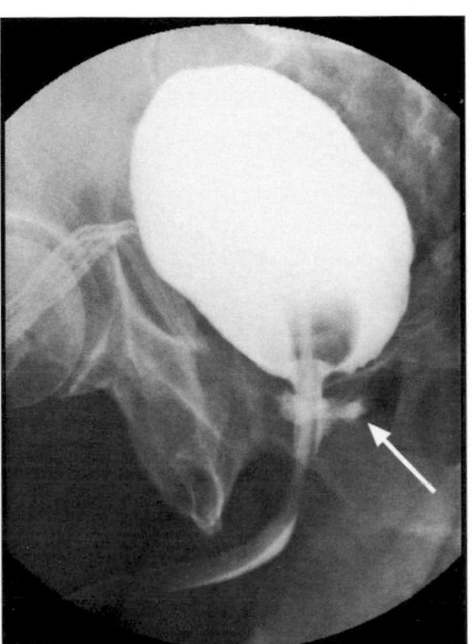

Fig. 2.25 Postoperative follow-up after prostatectomy. VCUG. Small extravasation at the anastomotic site (arrow).

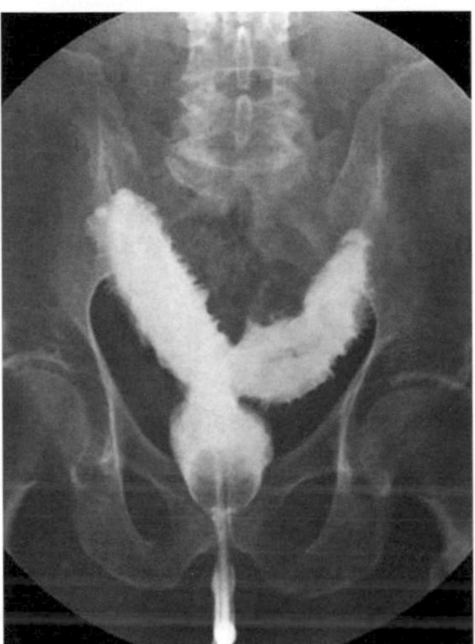

Fig. 2.26 Postoperative follow-up after creation of an ileal neobladder. VCUG. No extravasation. The contour of the bladder substitute corresponds to the small intestine.

Selected References

Beyersdorff D. Harnblase. In: Freyschmidt J et al (eds). Handbuch für Radiologie. Heidelberg: Springer; 2004

Dunnick NR et al (eds). Textbook of Uroradiology. The urinary bladder/Diverticula. Philadelphia: Lippincott Williams & Wilkins; 2001: 362–364

Definition

Extraperitoneal or intraperitoneal rupture of the urinary bladder • Combined extra- and intraperitoneal rupture in patients with complex injuries.

▸ **Etiology**

Blunt, penetrating, or iatrogenic trauma • Extraperitoneal rupture in 80–90% of cases • Bladder injury in a motor vehicle accident from the seatbelt when the bladder is full (blunt trauma) or from sharp bone fragments (pubic bone) in patients with pelvic fracture (penetrating trauma) • Risk of bladder injury increases with degree of bladder distention.

Imaging Signs

▸ **Modality of choice**

CT cystography.

▸ **Pathognomonic findings**

Extravasation of contrast medium contiguous with the bladder.

▸ **CT findings**

Tear in the bladder wall is often directly seen • Fluid outlining the bladder • Foreign body may be present in penetrating injury • Attenuation value of urine: 0–20 HU • Attenuation value of hemorrhage: 30–50 HU.

▸ **Cystographic findings**

Deformity or displacement of the bladder • Extraperitoneal extravasation with contrast medium in the perivesical soft tissues (including retroperitoneal space, scrotum, pelvic wall, perirenal tissue) or intraperitoneal extravasation (pouch of Douglas, interenteric).

Clinical Aspects

▸ **Typical presentation**

Suprapubic pain • Gross hematuria.

▸ **Treatment options**

Extraperitoneal rupture can be treated conservatively by antibiotics and catheterization • Suture repair in case of intraperitoneal rupture.

▸ **Course and prognosis**

Depend on severity • Small injuries may heal spontaneously • Risk of complications increases with the extent of injury (fistula, abscess, urinoma).

▸ **What does the clinician want to know?**

Presence of intraperitoneal rupture, which would require surgical intervention.

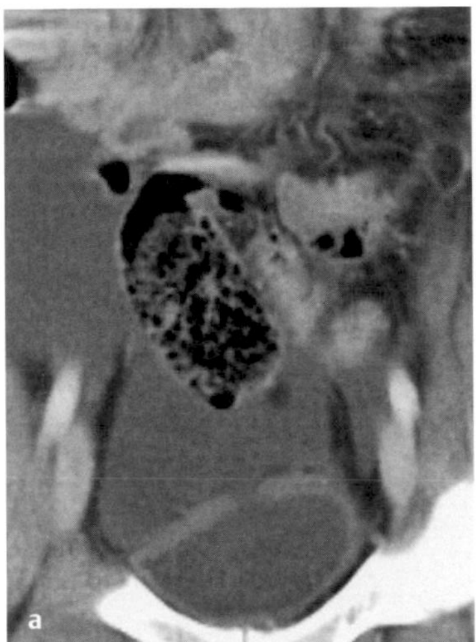

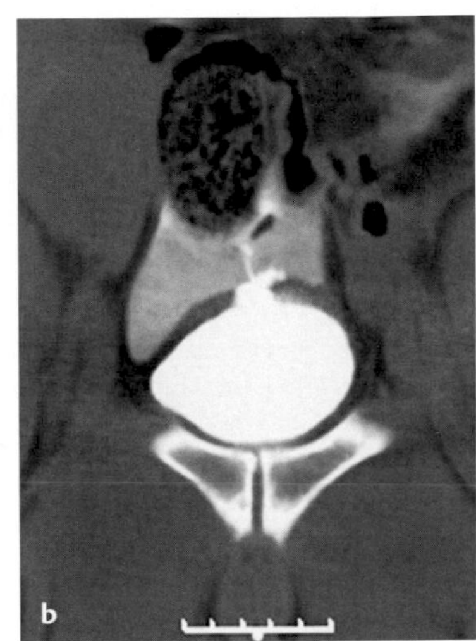

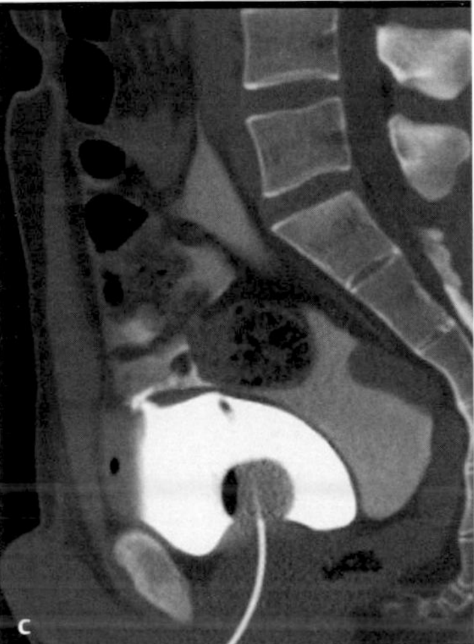

Fig. 2.27 a–c Intraperitoneal bladder rupture after a motor vehicle accident. CT.

a Coronal reconstruction. Circumscribed partial tear in the dome of the bladder.

b, c CT cystography. Intraperitoneal contrast extravasation from the bladder is diagnostic of bladder rupture (kindly provided by Prof. S. Mutze, MD, Unfallkrankenhaus Berlin).

Differential Diagnosis

Blood clot in the bladder	– No extravasation from the bladder
Hemoperitoneum	– Higher attenuation on CT
Retroperitoneal hematoma	– No extravasation from the bladder

Tips and Pitfalls

Bladder rupture is often overlooked if no late phase CT scan is obtained • *Cystography:* Postvoid film is mandatory because a filled bladder can mask extravasated contrast medium • Urethral injury must be excluded in trauma patients before inserting a transurethral catheter (or use suprapubic access).

Selected References

Morey AF et al. Bladder rupture after blunt trauma: guidelines for diagnostic imaging. J Trauma 2001; 51: 683–686

Peng MY et al. CT cystography versus conventional cystography in evaluation of bladder injury. AJR Am J Roentgenol 1999; 173: 1269–1272

Vaccaro JP, Brody JM. CT cystography in the evaluation of major bladder trauma. Radiographics 2000; 20: 1373–1381

Definition

- **Etiology**
  Accidents such as straddle injury • Rupture of the corpus cavernosum (penile fracture) due to blunt trauma to the erect penis during vigorous intercourse; may be associated with urethral injury • Iatrogenic injury, e.g., from urethral instrumentation.

Imaging Signs

- **Modality of choice**
  Retrograde urethrography • MRI to evaluate penile fracture.
- **Retrograde urethrographic findings**
  A retrograde urethrogram should be obtained in all trauma patients in whom urethral injury cannot be excluded, especially before bladder catheterization • Urethral injury is indicated by contrast extravasation or discontinuity.
- **MRI findings**
  MRI is indicated in patients with penile fracture • Imaging with a surface coil (e.g., loop coil) with the penis placed medially • Axial and sagittal T2-weighted TSE sequences and sagittal T1-weighted sequence • Slice thickness of 3 mm • Good visualization of the corpora cavernosa • Hypointense tunica albuginea • Penile fracture is depicted as discontinuity of the tunica albuginea • Often concomitant subcutaneous hematoma.
- **Ultrasound findings**
  Disrupted tunica albuginea • Ultrasound is less reliable than MRI.

Clinical Aspects

- **Typical presentation**
  History of trauma • Pain • Possible hematoma • Urinary retention requires prompt diagnosis because it is highly indicative of urethral injury.
- **Treatment options**
  Surgery in case of corpus cavernosum injury • Treatment of urethral injury varies with severity—suprapubic drainage of urine, urethral stent, surgery.
- **Course and prognosis**
  Corpus cavernosum injury can cause deviation and erectile dysfunction • Recurrent urethral strictures may occur after urethral injury.
- **What does the clinician want to know?**
  Presence of urethral injury/corpus cavernosum fracture • Site and extent of cavernosal injury.

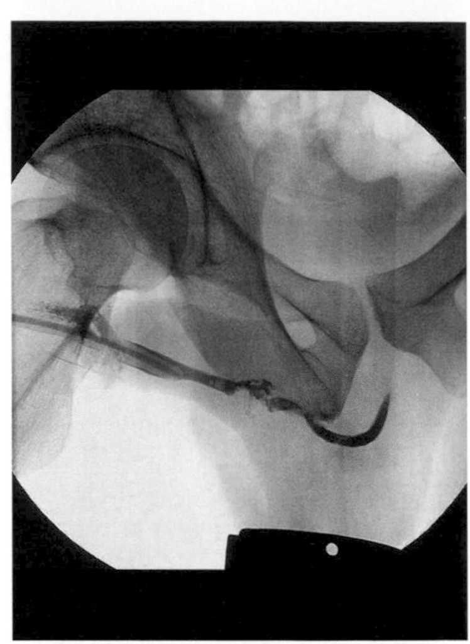

Fig. 2.28 Urethral injury. Retrograde urethrogram.

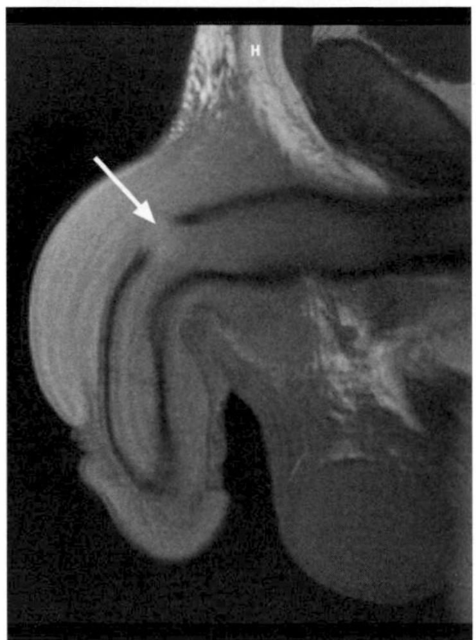

Fig. 2.29 Penile fracture. Sagittal T1-weighted MR image. Discontinuity of the hypointense tunica albuginea (arrow).

Differential Diagnosis

Subcutaneous hematoma	– Intact urethra and corpora cavernosa
Older urethral stricture	– Urethral narrowing without contrast extravasation – History

Tips and Pitfalls

Do not catheterize the bladder in patients with possible urethral injury before a retrograde urethrogram has been obtained.

Selected References

Bertolotto M et al. Imaging of penile traumas—therapeutic implications. Eur Radiol 2005; 15: 2475–2482

Kawashima A et al. Imaging of urethral disease: A pictorial review. Radiographics 2004; 24: S195–216

Definition

► **Anatomy**
Each testis consists of lobules containing densely packed convoluted seminiferous tubules • The straight terminal portions of the seminiferous tubules join to form the rete testis, enter the mediastinum testis, and become the efferent ductules • The ductules pierce through the tunica albuginea to form the head of epididymis and then converge into the larger vas deferens in the body and tail • The seminiferous tubules are composed of germ cells and Sertoli cells • Testosterone-producing Leydig cells are in the testicular interstitium • *Tunica albuginea:* this is a dense fibrous capsule with an overlying mesothelial layer, enclosing the testis.

Imaging Signs

► **Modality of choice**
Ultrasound • May be supplemented by MRI.

► **Ultrasound findings**
Testis: Ovoid organ • Size: 4–5 × 2–3 × 2–2.5 cm • Volume: 15–20 mL • Intermediate echogenicity and fine granular echotexture • *Infant testis:* 1.5 × 1 cm in size and of lower echogenicity • Small amount of serous fluid should not be misinterpreted as hydrocele.
Tunica albuginea: Thin echogenic line surrounding the testis • Best seen where it reflects into the testis as the mediastinum testis.
Mediastinum testis: Echogenic • Located eccentrically • Tubules coursing in a caudocranial direction.
Scrotal cavity: Thin anechoic rim representing fluid is often seen, especially in the area adjacent to the head of epididymis.
Epididymis: Isoechoic or hypoechoic and somewhat coarser than the testis • Pyramidal head at the upper pole of the testis, 5–12 mm in length • Width of the body lateral to the testis: 2–4 mm • Width of the tail at the lower pole: 2–5 mm.
Epididymal appendix: Pedunculated hydatid attached to the epididymal head.
Testicular appendix (hydatid of Morgagni): Ovoid hydatid, 5 mm in size, between the upper pole of the testis and the epididymis • Isoechoic • Cystic • Typically seen only when a hydrocele is present or in case of torsion.
Testicular artery: Primary vascular supply to the testis • Branch of the abdominal aorta • Pierces the tunica albuginea at the mediastinum, forming capsular arteries • Capsular arteries give off centripetal branches • An occasional variant runs directly within the mediastinum as a transmediastinal artery • RI 0.48–0.75.
Further arteries: Cremasteric artery (from the inferior epigastric artery) and deferential artery (from the vesical artery) • Supply the epididymis, vas deferens, and peritesticular tissue • RI 0.63–1.0.
Pampiniform plexus: Venous drainage • Part of the spermatic cord • Opens into the ipsilateral testicular vein.

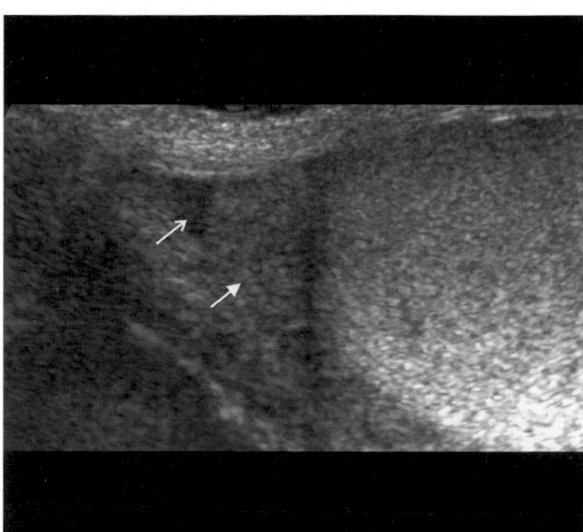

Fig. 3.1 Normal upper pole of the testis. Longitudinal ultrasound scan. Higher echogenicity of the testis in the polar region compared with the adjacent pyramidal head of the epididymis (filled arrow). A small amount of fluid in the scrotum (open arrow) is normal.

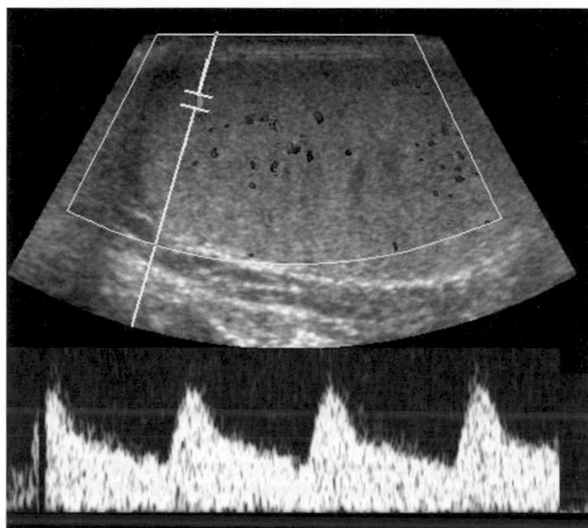

Fig. 3.2 Doppler ultrasound of the testis. Normal biphasic arterial flow pattern.

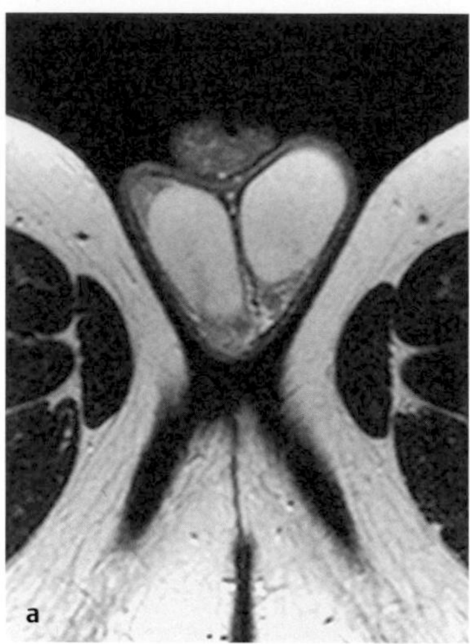

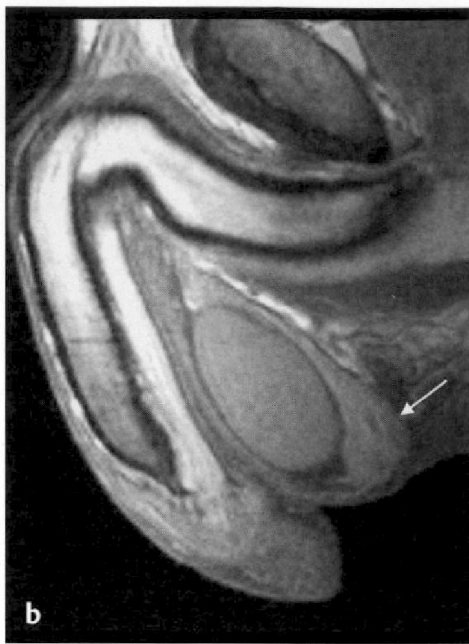

Fig. 3.3 a, b Normal testes. MR images.

a Axial T2-weighted image. Testes with normal high signal intensity.

b Sagittal T1-weighted image after intravenous contrast administration. Testis with intermediate signal intensity. Normal tail of epididymis (arrow).

► **MRI findings**

Testis: Homogeneous intermediate signal intensity on T1-weighted images • High signal intensity on T2-weighted images • Hypointense septa radially extending from the capsule to the mediastinum testis • *Tunica albuginea:* Thin line of low signal intensity.

Epididymis: Isointense to testis on T1-weighted images, hypointense on T2-weighted images • More marked contrast enhancement compared with the testis.

Differential Diagnosis

Cryptorchidism	– Undescended testis, seen in 3% of newborns, may descend spontaneously in the first year of life – Inguinal testes are followed up by ultrasound, abdominal testes by MRI – Persistent undescended testis will atrophy and has a higher risk of testicular tumor

Selected References

Hricak H et al. Imaging of the Scrotum. New York: Raven Press; 1995

Definition

- **Epidemiology**
  Most common cause of painless scrotal swelling.
- **Etiology**
  Excessive accumulation of serous fluid in the scrotum • *Congenital:* Patent processus vaginalis (communication with the abdominal cavity) in newborns • Resolves spontaneously within the first year of life • *Spermatic cord hydrocele:* Small fluid collection due to incomplete closure of the processus vaginalis • *Acquired:* Reactive hydrocele due to inguinal hernia, epididymoorchitis, vascular obstruction, trauma, or ascites • Idiopathic hydrocele.

Imaging Signs

- **Modality of choice**
  Ultrasound.
- **Ultrasound findings**
  Anechoic crescent-shaped fluid collection around the testis and epididymis • Septa and scrotal wall thickening in chronic inflammatory hydrocele • Internal echoes indicate high protein content • Hydrocele may contain scrotoliths (scrotal pearls) seen as small echogenic calculi with posterior shadowing.

Clinical Aspects

- **Typical presentation**
  Painless swelling and soft fullness within the scrotum • The underlying testis cannot be palpated.
- **Treatment options**
  Treatment of the underlying cause • Fenestration and plication of the tunica vaginalis • Tetracycline sclerotherapy • Expectant management in newborns.
- **What does the clinician want to know?**
  Exclusion of a testicular tumor.

Differential Diagnosis

Pyocele	– Floating echoes within the fluid – Signs of inflammation
Hematocele	– History of trauma – Acute hematocele is more echogenic – Organized hematocele is more complex and heterogeneous

Selected References

Hricak H et al. Imaging of the Scrotum. New York: Raven Press; 1995

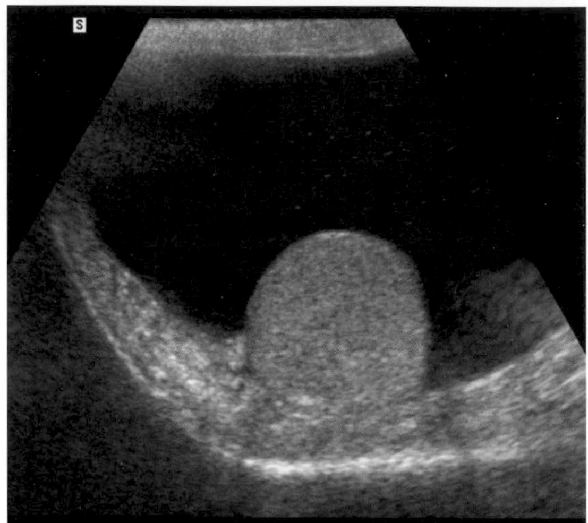

Fig. 3.4 Hydrocele. Transverse ultrasound scan showing large hydrocele surrounding the left testis.

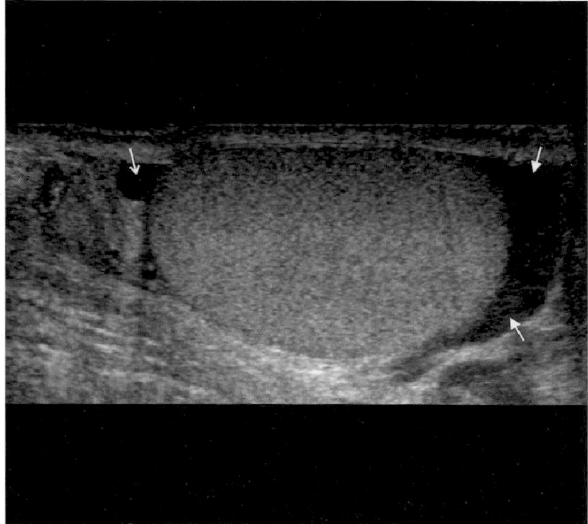

Fig. 3.5 Small hydrocele. Longitudinal ultrasound scan of the right testis. Anechoic band around the inferior pole of the testis (filled arrows). Accessory finding: spermatocele in the epididymal head (open arrow).

Definition

- **Epidemiology**
  Present in 10% of men • Mostly spermatoceles • True epididymal and intratesticular cysts are rare • Tunica albuginea cysts are more common • Cystic transformation of the rete testis (tubular ectasia), typically caused by obliteration of the efferent ducts in older men.
- **Etiology**
  Spermatocele: Cystic distention of the efferent ducts in the epididymis • True cysts may occur anywhere in the epididymis • Testicular cysts in older men.

Imaging Signs

- **Modality of choice**
  Ultrasound.
- **Ultrasound findings**
  Spermatocele: Thin-walled anechoic cyst, only occurring in the epididymal head • Posterior acoustic enhancement • Single or multilocular • May contain internal echoes • Septa and sediments in rare cases • Cannot be differentiated from a true cyst in the epididymal head.
  Testicular cysts and tunica albuginea cysts: Intratesticular cysts located near the mediastinum testis • Tunica albuginea cysts are subcapsular in location • Thin-walled • Normal echotexture of surrounding testicular parenchyma • Rare.
  Tubular ectasia of the rete testis: Anechoic tubules and cysts are seen side by side in the mediastinum testis.

Clinical Aspects

- **Typical presentation**
  Spermatoceles cause no symptoms • Intratesticular cysts not palpable • Tunica albuginea cysts palpable as focal masses • Large cysts may cause a dragging sensation.
- **Treatment options**
  No treatment required.
- **What does the clinician want to know?**
  Differential diagnosis, especially of intratesticular cysts and testicular tumors.

Differential Diagnosis

Testicular tumors	– Especially nonseminomas with cystic components – Solid tumor components and palpable mass
Adenomatoid tumor	– Solid benign tumor of the tail of epididymis

Selected References

Hricak H et al. Imaging of the Scrotum. New York: Raven Press; 1995

Fig. 3.6 Diagrammatic representation of testicular and epididymal cysts.

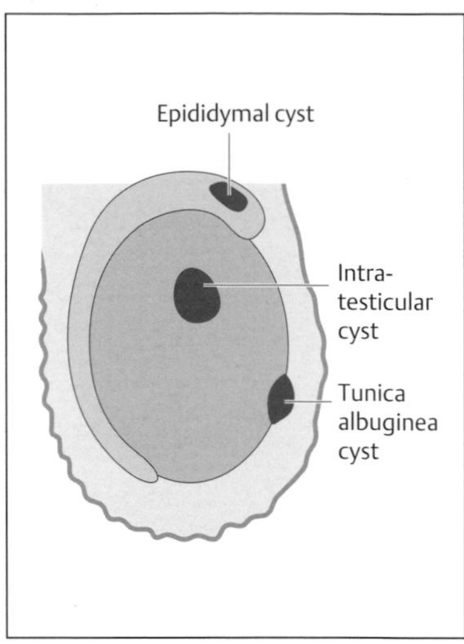

Fig. 3.7 Longitudinal scan of the right testis. Doppler ultrasound. Anechoic spermatocele in the epididymal head (arrow).

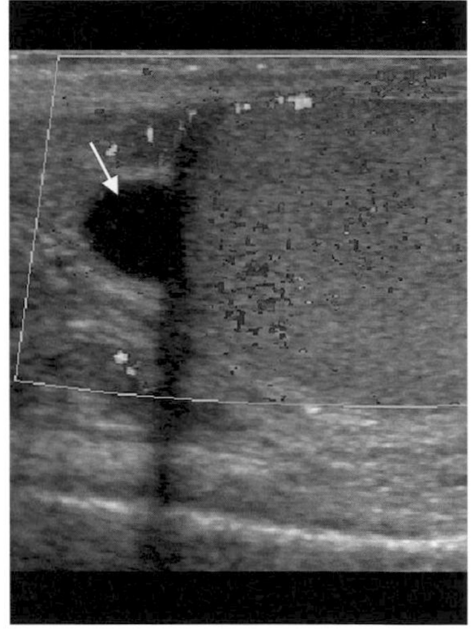

Definition

- **Epidemiology**
  Prevalence of up to 9% in the USA • Association with testicular tumors, especially germ cell tumors.
- **Etiology**
  Calcifications of the seminiferous tubules • Unclear etiology.

Imaging Signs

- **Modality of choice**
  Ultrasound.
- **Ultrasound findings**
  Multiple hyperechoic foci in both testicles (diagnostic criterion: more than five microliths on at least one ultrasound image) • 1–2 mm in size • Diffuse distribution • No posterior shadowing • Incidental finding.

Clinical Aspects

- **Typical presentation**
  Asymptomatic.
- **Treatment options**
  Some centers recommend annual sonographic follow-up to rule out tumor.
- **What does the clinician want to know?**
  Exclusion of a testicular tumor.

Differential Diagnosis

Macrocalcifications of the testis	– After trauma – Teratoma, Sertoli cell tumor – Burned-out tumor
Other macrocalcifications	– Tunica albuginea plaque after trauma – Epididymal calcifications after granulomatous inflammation (tuberculosis) or trauma – Scrotoliths (scrotal pearls) within the scrotum

Selected References

Hricak H et al. Imaging of the Scrotum. New York: Raven Press; 1995

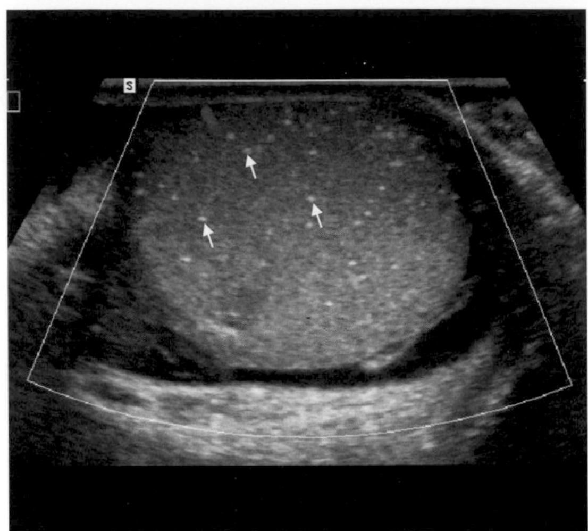

Fig. 3.8 Longitudinal ultrasound scan of the left testis. Testicular microlithiasis is indicated by the numerous echogenic foci scattered throughout the testis. Three punctate calcifications are indicated by arrows.

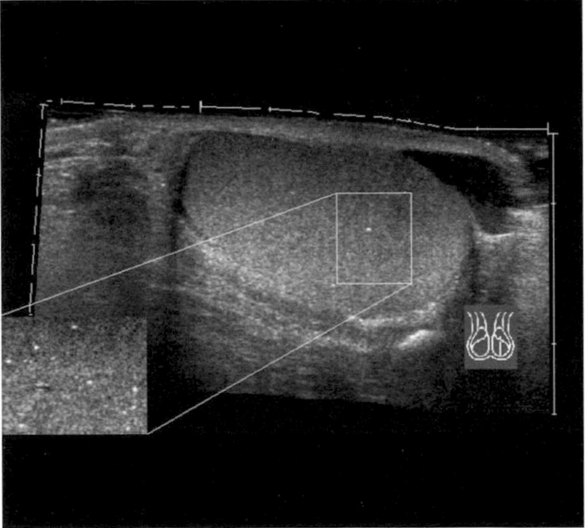

Fig. 3.9 Longitudinal ultrasound scan of the right testis. Testicular microlithiasis is apparent only after magnification.

Definition

- **Epidemiology**
  Epididymitis is the most common cause of acute scrotum • Concomitant orchitis in 20% of patients with epididymitis • Isolated orchitis is rare, and most cases are due to mumps.
- **Etiology**
  Nonspecific bacterial infection • Ascending spread via the vas deferens, e.g., in urethritis or prostatitis • Granulomatous epididymitis in sarcoidosis, tuberculosis, syphilis, leprosy.

Imaging Signs

- **Modality of choice**
  Ultrasound.
- **Ultrasound findings**
  Acute stage: Enlargement of the entire epididymis and testis or predominantly the epididymal tail in less severe forms • Coarser and more hypoechoic echotexture • Diffuse or focal (primarily at the upper pole of the testis) • Reactive hydrocele.
  Pyocele: Internal echoes • Scrotal wall thickening • Hypervascularization • RI often < 0.5, $V_{max} > 15$ cm/s.
  Granulomatous epididymitis/orchitis: Hypoechoic nodules with hypervascular rim • Virtually impossible to differentiate from tumor.
  Epididymitis nodosa: Chronic • Cystic inclusions.
  Abscess: Hypoechoic lesion with irregular borders • Internal echoes • Hypervascular rim.

Clinical Aspects

- **Typical presentation**
  Gradual increase in pain • Pain becomes more severe with pressure and movement • Positive Prehn sign—scrotal elevation and support relieves pain • Testicular swelling • Fever.
  Complications: Abscess formation • Fistula • Infarction • Infertility, e.g., due to occlusive azoospermia • Testicular atrophy • Sterility.
- **Treatment options**
  Identification of the causative microorganism • Antibiotic treatment • Anti-inflammatory treatment • Surgery if there are complications.
- **What does the clinician want to know?**
  Differential diagnosis of acute scrotum (torsion, exclusion of tumor).

Fig. 3.10 a, b Epididymoorchitis. Ultrasound.

a Longitudinal scan of the left testis and epididymis. Enlargement and coarser echotexture of the epididymis (arrows).

b Hypervascularization. Small hydrocele (asterisk).

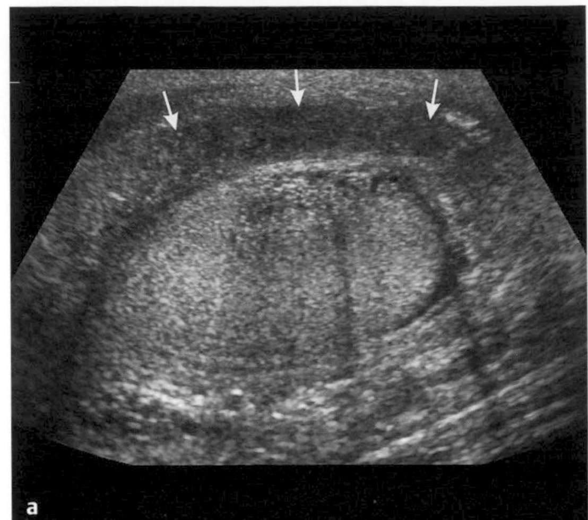

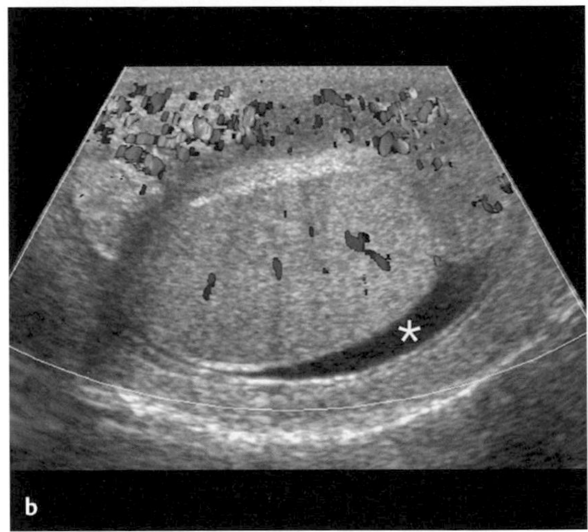

Differential Diagnosis

Testicular torsion	– No hypervascularization – Increased RI
Testicular tumor	– Focal intratesticular tumor – Biopsy to differentiate testicular tumor from chronic focal orchitis in unclear cases

Selected References

Hricak H et al. Imaging of the Scrotum. New York: Raven Press; 1995

Definition

▸ **Epidemiology**

Represent 1% of all neoplasms in men • Most common solid neoplasms in men between 15 and 40 years.

▸ **Histology**

Malignant germ cell tumors: 90% of all testicular tumors.

- Seminoma: Peak age 36 years, 35%.
- Nonseminomas: Peak age 26 years • Embryonal carcinoma, 20% • Teratoma, 25% • Mixed tumors, 15% • Choriocarcinoma, less than 1%.
- Burned-out tumor: Regressed testicular tumor with metastatic spread.

Stromal tumors: 5% of all testicular tumors • Leydig cell tumors and less commonly Sertoli cell tumors • 90% are benign • Occur at any age • Frequently associated with abnormal sexual development.

Nonprimary testicular tumors:

- Lymphoma: Especially in men aged 60 or older • Usually B-cell NHL • 5% of all testicular tumors • Typical manifestation of recurrent leukemia after chemotherapy in children (blood–testis barrier).
- Metastasis: Rare • Typically from prostate or bronchial cancer.

▸ **Etiology**

Risk factors: Undescended testis, microlithiasis, contralateral testicular tumor.

Imaging Signs

▸ **Modality of choice**

Ultrasound • MRI • CT to exclude metastasis.

▸ **Ultrasound findings**

Focal intratesticular lesion • Irregularity in the normal homogeneous, medium-level echotexture of the testis • Large tumors completely replace the testis or leave only a thin margin of normal parenchyma • Sonographic findings must be correlated with palpation in all cases • Concomitant hydrocele may be present.

Local tumor staging by ultrasound is unreliable:

- T1: confined to the testis.
- T2: involves the tunica albuginea or the epididymis.
- T3: involves the spermatic cord.
- T4: involves the scrotum.

Tumor tissue types cannot be reliably differentiated solely by their ultrasonographic appearance and only histologic examination allows tumor characterization.

Seminoma: Hypoechoic • Smooth margins • Cystic components may be present • Hypervascular tumor.

Germ cell tumors: Heterogeneous • Calcifications • Fibrosis • Contain cartilage, bone, and cysts • Irregular contour • Invasion of the tunica albuginea.

Teratoma: Heterogeneous • Macrocalcifications • Complex cysts (internal echoes, thickened wall, septa).

Burned-out tumor: Echogenic scar or calcification • No focal lesion.

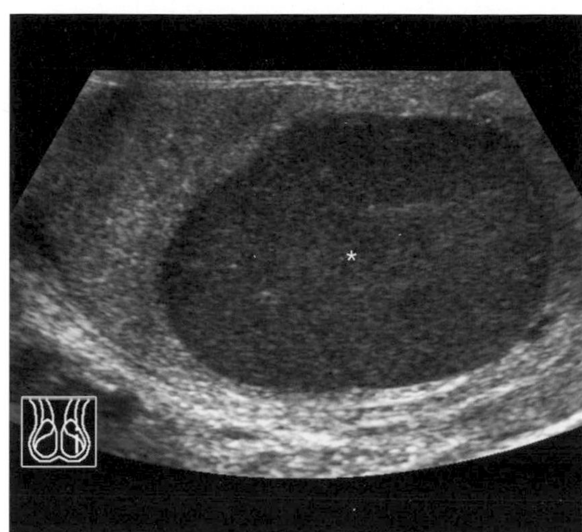

Fig. 3.11 Seminoma in a 42-year-old man presenting with a palpable mass. Longitudinal ultrasound scan of the left testis. Large, hypoechoic, smoothly marginated mass (asterisk) in the left testis.

Sertoli cell tumor: Hypoechoic • Smoothly marginated • Round • Lobulated.
Leydig cell tumor: Cystic • Necrotic • Hemorrhagic • Small.
Lymphoma/leukemia: Hypoechoic • One or multiple lesions • Testicular enlargement • Geographic echopattern • Often bilateral • Hypervascular • Involvement of the epididymis and spermatic cord.

- **MRI findings**
Hypointense mass on T2-weighted images, isointense to hypointense on T1-weighted images • Inhomogeneous areas due to calcifications, necrosis, and hemorrhage.
- **CT findings**
Detection of retroperitoneal lymph node and lung metastases, if present.

Clinical Aspects

- **Typical presentation**
Painless, palpable mass • Testicular enlargement • Most testicular tumors are discovered by the patients themselves • 10% present with acute pain and fever • Hormonally active stromal tumors cause bilateral gynecomastia, precocious virilization, and loss of libido • Lymphoma is associated with weight loss and often bilateral testicular swelling.

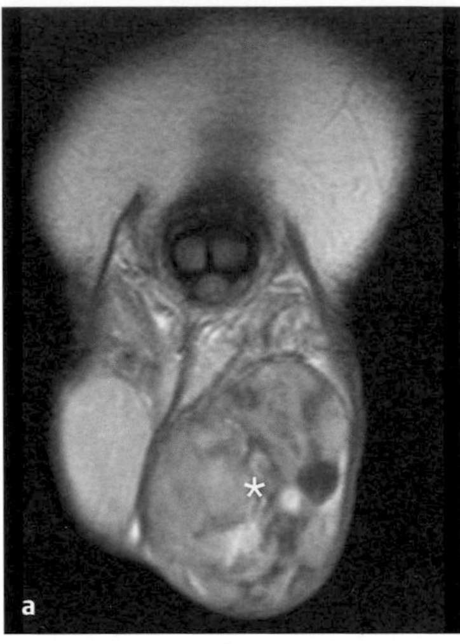

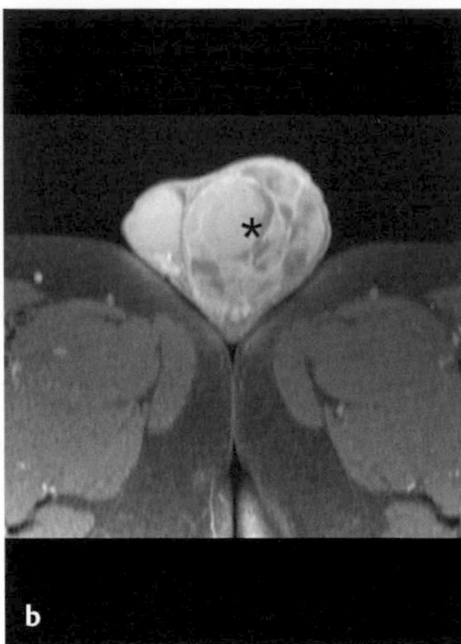

Fig. 3.12 a, b Nonseminoma in left testis. MR images. Mass (asterisks) with liquid inclusions. Normal right testis.
a Coronal T2-weighted image.
b Axial contrast-enhanced T1-weighted image with fat saturation.

► **Course**
- *Stage I:* No metastases.
- *Stage II:* Lymph node metastases below the diaphragm.
- *Stage III:* Lymph node metastases above the diaphragm.

Germ cell tumors: Lymphatic spread to retroperitoneal, paraaortic, and supraclavicular lymph nodes • Late hematogenous spread, e.g., to the lungs • Choriocarcinoma is an exception with early hematogenous spread typically to the brain.

► **Treatment options**

Orchiectomy • Adjuvant prophylactic retroperitoneal radiotherapy in seminoma • Abdominal lymph node dissection in patients with nonseminoma and suspected lymph node involvement • Possible adjuvant chemotherapy, e.g., in patients with lymphatic metastatic spread of nonseminoma • Neoadjuvant chemotherapy with subsequent resection in advanced testicular cancer.

► **Prognosis**
- *Seminoma:* 100% 5-year survival rate in stage I, 85% in metastatic seminoma.
- *Nonseminoma:* 100% 5-year survival rate in stage I, 95% in tumors with retroperitoneal metastases, and 30% in the presence of distant metastases.
- *Choriocarcinoma:* Very poor 1-year survival rate.

► **What does the clinician want to know?**

Differentiation of palpable scrotal masses—intratesticular versus extratesticular.

Differential Diagnosis

Epidermoid/keratocyst	– Benign, smoothly marginated, round focal lesion 1–3 cm in size – Typically between 20 and 40 years of age – Target or onion ring appearance (concentric rings of hypo- and hyperechogenicity) – Not vascularized – Wall calcifications are rare – Treatment—enucleation
Focal orchitis, granulomatous orchitis	– One or multiple hypoechoic intratesticular areas – Most patients have signs of concomitant epididymitis – Chronic form is difficult to distinguish from tumor
Abscess	– Complication of epididymoorchitis or after trauma – Hypoechoic, irregular lesion with internal echoes and hypervascular rim
Infarction	– Complication of epididymoorchitis or in older men – Hypoechoic lesion – Decreases in size over time
Marchand rests	– Very rare – Hyperplasia of normal testicular adrenal rests (which are present in 10% of men) due to congenital adrenal hyperplasia and Cushing syndrome – Multiple, heterogeneous, hypoechoic lesions in both testes – Hypointense lesions on T1- and T2-weighted MRI – Treatment—hormone replacement

Tips and Pitfalls

Always palpate the mass.

Selected References

Hricak H et al. Imaging of the Scrotum. New York: Raven Press; 1995

Woodward PJ et al. From the archives of the AFIP. Tumors and tumorlike lesions of the testis: radiologic-pathologic correlation. RadioGraphics 2002; 22: 189–216

Definition

Urologic emergency • Rotation of the testis on the spermatic cord with subsequent ischemia • Rotation of less than 360° initially only obstructs venous drainage • Rotation of more than 360° (complete torsion) additionally compromises arterial inflow and causes ischemia • Extravaginal torsion with rotation involving the testis and its coverings in newborns • Intravaginal testicular torsion in older boys and adult men.

- **Epidemiology**
  Testicular pain accounts for 0.5% of emergency presentations.

Imaging Signs

- **Modality of choice**
  Ultrasound.
- **Ultrasound findings**
  Ultrasound is performed using a linear transducer with at least 7.5 MHz and color/pulsed-wave Doppler capabilities • A twisted spermatic cord is seen in most cases • Focal distention and inhomogeneous echotexture of the spermatic cord with anechoic, spiral tubular structures (representing the rotated vessels) • Reduced testicular perfusion • Increased resistance with RI > 0.75 or to-and-fro flow • Complete absence of testicular flow with rotation > 360° • B-mode ultrasound shows no changes of the testicular parenchyma within the first hours of onset • Swelling and diffuse hypoechoic changes seen later • Inhomogeneous or striated echotexture of the testis after 24 hours.

Clinical Aspects

- **Typical presentation**
  Clinically, it is often not possible to differentiate between testicular torsion, hydatid torsion, epididymitis, and orchitis in patients presenting with testicular pain • Testicular torsion can occur at any age but is most common in adolescents • Typically acute onset of pain with no relief on scrotal elevation.
- **Treatment options**
  Surgical exploration is necessary in all unclear cases • Ipsilateral and contralateral orchiopexy in patients with surgically confirmed testicular torsion, because the bell clapper deformity (tunica vaginalis completely surrounding the testis), which predisposes to testicular torsion, is usually bilateral.
- **Course and prognosis**
  Spontaneous detorsion may occur • The rate of testicular salvage is nearly 100% if treatment is performed within the first 6 hours, 50% within 6–12 hours, and 20% within 12–24 hours.
- **What does the clinician want to know?**
  Exclusion of testicular torsion in patients with acute testicular pain.

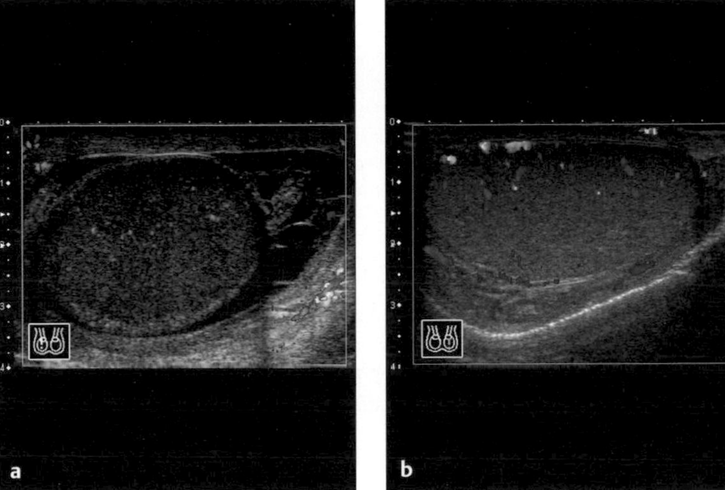

Fig. 3.13 a, b Testicular torsion. Ultrasound.
a No flow in the testicular vessels. Perfusion only in the vessels near the scrotal wall.
b Normal perfusion of the contralateral testis.

Differential Diagnosis

Epididymitis	– Hyperemia of the epididymis
Partial torsion	– Preserved arterial flow, increased RI
Orchitis	– Hyperemia of the testicular parenchyma
Appendage torsion	– Enlarged appendage at the upper pole of the testis – Firm, with surrounding hyperemia – Typically occurs between 7 and 14 years

Tips and Pitfalls

Ultrasound should include color or pulsed-wave Doppler.

Selected References

Kraychick S et al. Color Doppler sonography: its real role in the evaluation of children with highly suspected testicular torsion. European Radiology 2001; 11: 1000–1005

Lesnik G et al. Sonographie des Skrotalinhalts. Fortschr Röntgenstr 2006; 178: 165–179

Definition

- **Etiology**
  Often blunt testicular trauma (e.g., sports injuries, motor vehicle accidents) • Stab and gunshot wounds • Surgery • Spontaneous intratesticular hemorrhage under anticoagulant treatment • Mobility renders testes less susceptible to injury • Testicular rupture is uncommon because the testis is protected by the strong tunica albuginea • Trauma is a rare cause of testicular torsion.

Imaging Signs

- **Modality of choice**
  Ultrasound.
- **Ultrasound findings**
  - *Testicular rupture:* Discontinuity of the tunica albuginea with extrusion of testicular tissue and concomitant edema • Heterogeneous testicular parenchyma.
  - *Testicular fragmentation:* Shattering of the testis.
  - *Testicular contusion:* Heterogeneous testicular echotexture due to hemorrhage.
  - *Scrotal edema:* Thickening of the scrotal coverings.
  - *Scrotal hematocele:* Hyperechoic in the acute stage • Organizing hematocele becomes heterogeneously hypoechoic with septa and blood–fluid levels.
  - *Testicular hematoma:* Intraparenchymal • Subcapsular.
  - *Peritesticular hematoma:* Involves the epididymis and scrotal coverings • Variable echogenicity (acute: hyperechoic; older hematoma: heterogeneous, cystic septa, fluid levels) • No perfusion.
  - *Posttraumatic testicular scars:* Hypoechoic • Irregular bands • Sharply delineated.
- **MRI findings**
  Signal intensities of intrascrotal and intratesticular hemorrhage:
  - First 24 hours: Intermediate signal intensity on T1-weighted images • Moderately hyperintense on T2-weighted images.
  - 24 hours to 3 days: Hypointense on T1- and T2-weighted images.
  - 3 to 7 days: Hyperintense on T1-weighted images • Hypointense on T2-weighted images.
  - 7 days to 2 weeks: Hyperintense on T1- and T2-weighted images.
  - After 2 weeks: Intermediate to low signal on T1- and T2-weighted images.

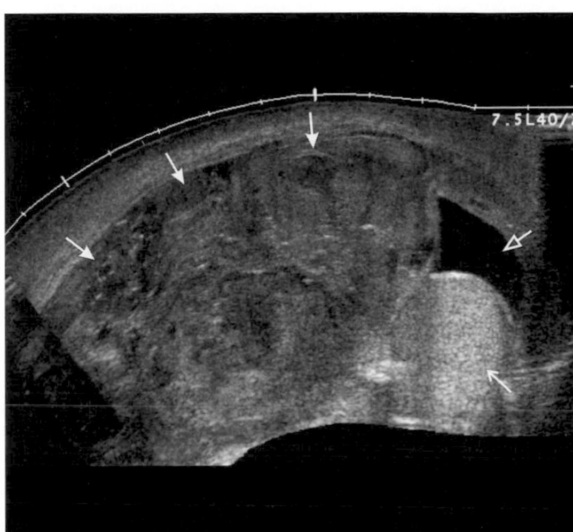

Fig. 3.14 Testicular trauma. Transverse ultrasound scan of the left scrotum. Partially organized scrotal hematoma (filled arrows) after trauma. Small hydrocele (empty arrow). Normal testis (open arrow).

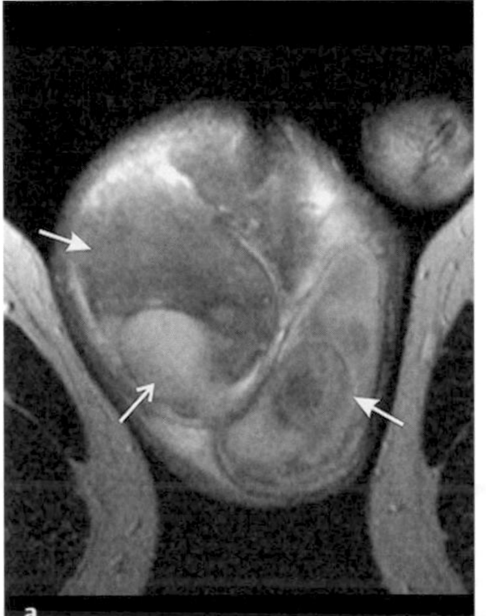

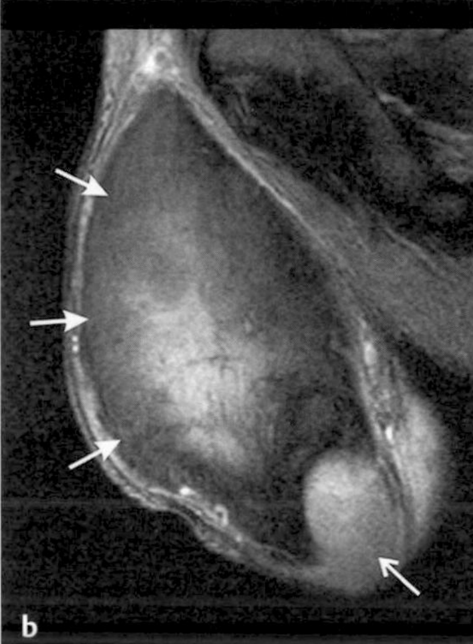

Fig. 3.15 a, b Iatrogenic testicular trauma. MR images. Large scrotal hematoma of heterogeneous signal intensity (filled arrows) after testicular biopsy. Normal testis on the right (open arrows).

a Axial T2-weighted image.

b Sagittal T2-weighted image.

Clinical Aspects

- **Typical presentation**
  Acute scrotum • Swelling • Induration • Severe pain • Avulsion of the scrotal skin.
- **Course**
  Varies with severity • Resolution with scar formation • Possible testicular atrophy.
- **Treatment options**
  Small hematoma is managed conservatively • Surgical exploration and drainage in case of large hematoma • Surgical management of testicular rupture • Possible hemicastration • Wound debridement • Elevation and cooling of the testis after surgery.
- **Prognosis**
  Depends on severity but good in most cases.
- **What does the clinician want to know?**
  Sequelae of trauma • Presence of testicular rupture • Follow-up findings.

Differential Diagnosis

Testicular tumor	– 10% of testicular tumors become symptomatic in association with trauma – A tumor persists while trauma-related changes resolve

Tips and Pitfalls

It is important to follow up traumatic intratesticular lesions until they have completely resolved to rule out testicular tumor.

Selected References

Hricak H et al. Imaging of the Scrotum. New York: Raven Press; 1995

Definition

A varicose condition of the veins of the pampiniform plexus due to reversal of flow from the internal spermatic vein • Affects only the left side in 80–90% of cases • Secondary varicocele due to compression of venous drainage in the retroperitoneum or along the spermatic vein, e.g., by renal cell carcinoma.

Imaging Signs

▸ **Modality of choice**
Ultrasound.

▸ **Routine diagnostic workup**
Inspection and palpation: In severe varicocele, the dilated veins appear bluish through the scrotal skin • Feels like a "bag of worms" with the patient standing • A primary varicocele often disappears when the patient lies down.
Venography: Time-consuming and invasive • Now largely replaced by ultrasound • Useful for performing retrograde sclerotherapy in the same session.

▸ **Ultrasound findings**
Ultrasound is carried out using a linear transducer with at least 7.5 MHz and color/pulsed-wave Doppler capabilities • Bilateral examination of the spermatic cord and testis • Varicose veins are easily identified • Diameter of normal pampiniform plexus veins is less than 2 mm • Larger veins identified by ultrasound before they become palpable suggest varicocele • Retrograde flow for over 1 s with Valsalva maneuver is indicative of varicocele • Possible atrophy of the ipsilateral testis.

Clinical Aspects

▸ **Typical presentation**
Usually asymptomatic • Dragging sensation in some cases • Severe forms already become apparent in boys • A varicocele is often diagnosed in men presenting with fertility problems (reduced fertility even with unilateral varicocele).

▸ **Course and prognosis**
Primary varicocele: Antegrade sclerotherapy, resection of the affected veins, or retrograde sclerotherapy • Occasional recurrence due to incomplete occlusion or collateral flow, e.g., via cremasteric vein.

▸ **What does the clinician want to know?**
Confirmation of the diagnosis • Associated testicular changes?

Differential Diagnosis

Secondary varicocele	– Cause of impaired venous drainage, e.g., retroperitoneal tumor or thrombosis

Tips and Pitfalls

As a varicocele may disappear in the supine position, ultrasound should be done during Valsalva maneuver and repeated with the patient standing if the findings

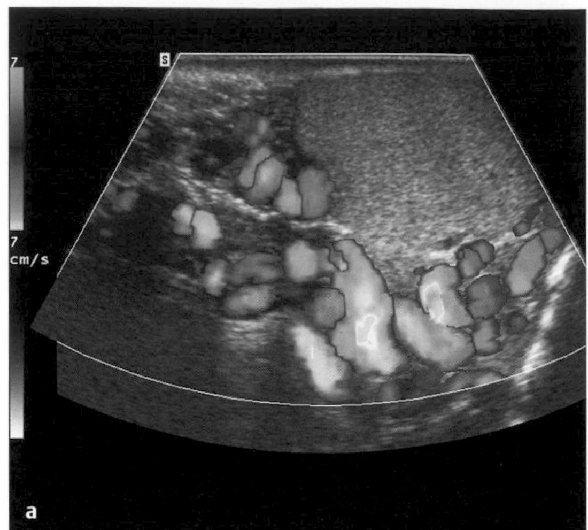

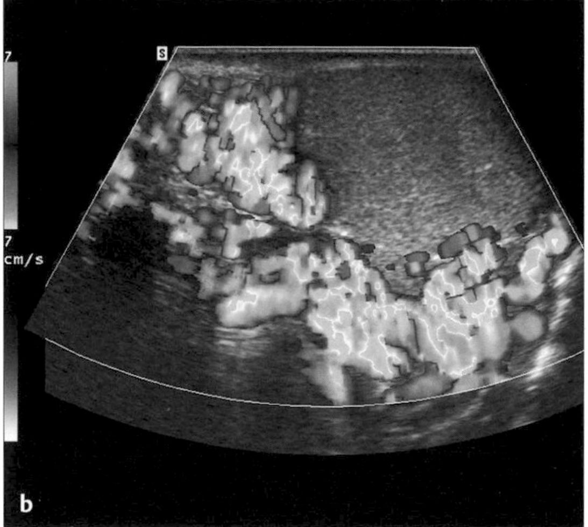

Fig. 3.16 a, b Varicocele. Ultrasound.
a Dilated veins of the spermatic cord.
b Retrograde flow during Valsalva maneuver.

are inconclusive • Exclude secondary varicocele in cases of recurrence and acute onset in adults.

Selected References

Beddy P et al. Testicular varicoceles. Clin Radiol 2005; 60: 1248–1255
Lesnik G et al. Sonographie des Skrotalinhalts. Fortschr Röntgenstr 2006; 178: 165–179

Definition

BPH is the adenomatous enlargement of the transitional zone of the prostate • It is a common condition that is considered abnormal when it causes bladder outlet obstruction and voiding problems • BPH is rarely the primary site of prostate cancer.

- **Epidemiology**
  Common in men aged 50 and older • Often progressive enlargement.

Imaging Signs

- **Modality of choice**
  Transrectal or transvesical ultrasound.
- **Routine diagnostic workup**
  Digital rectal examination • Transrectal or transvesical ultrasound is the first-line imaging modality • Retrograde urethrogram to rule out further urethral strictures in patients with bladder outlet obstruction.
- **Ultrasound findings**
  Inhomogeneous area of high and low echogenicity in the center of the prostate • Acoustic shadowing indicates calcifications • Limited visualization of prostate zonal anatomy.
- **Intravenous pyelogram findings**
  Protrusion of the enlarged prostate gland at the floor of the bladder • Significant enlargement of the prostate can cause bladder base elevation with "J-ing" or "fish hooking" of the distal ureters.
- **MRI findings**
  Exquisite visualization of the zonal anatomy on T2-weighted images • Well-defined enlarged transitional zone • Usually inhomogeneous with areas of high and low signal intensity • Smooth interface with the peripheral zone.
- **CT findings**
  No visualization of the zonal anatomy • Enlargement of the entire prostate gland • Median lobe protrudes into the floor of the bladder • Prostate cancer cannot be excluded.

Clinical Aspects

- **Typical presentation**
  Voiding problems • Reduced urine flow • Often detected in patients undergoing diagnostic assessment for PSA elevation or as an incidental finding on abdominal ultrasound.
- **Treatment options**
  Surgical adenectomy or TURP.
- **Course and prognosis**
  Excellent prognosis • Recurrent BPH is uncommon.
- **What does the clinician want to know?**
  Extent of BPH • Other causes of bladder outlet obstruction (e.g., urethral stricture)? • Signs of prostate cancer?

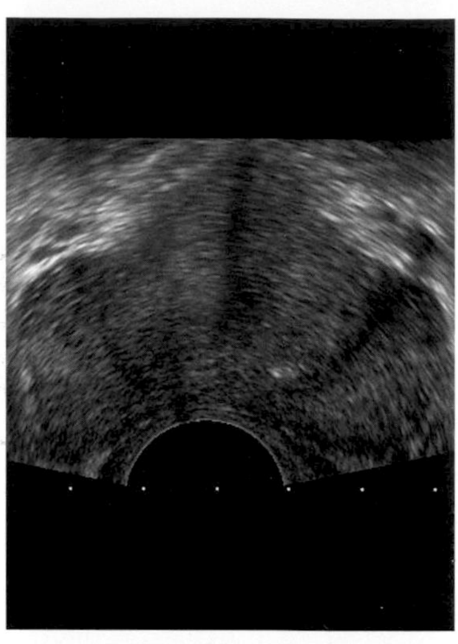

Fig. 3.17 Benign prostatic hyperplasia. Ultrasound.

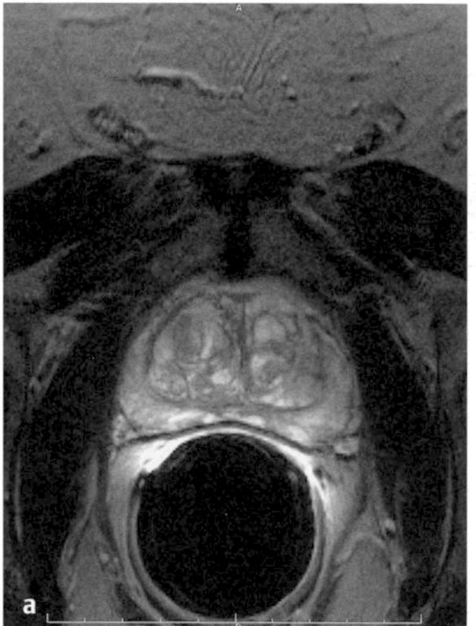

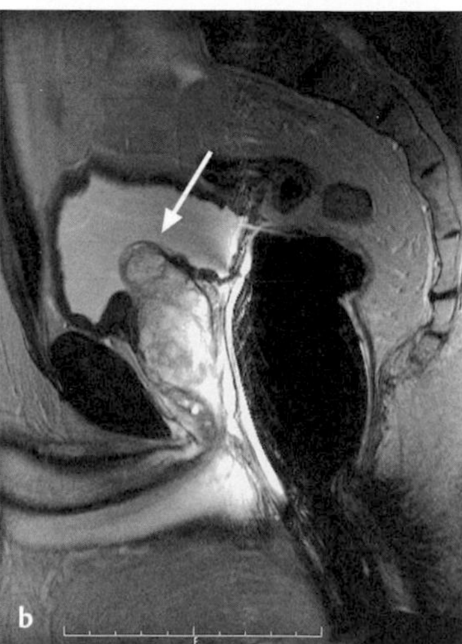

Fig. 3.18 a, b T2-weighted MRI sequence. Good visualization of the zonal anatomy of the prostate. The transitional zone is markedly enlarged and protrudes into the bladder base.

a Axial image.

b Sagittal image.

Differential Diagnosis

Prostate cancer	– Mainly in the peripheral zone of the prostate – Less bulbous – Biopsy to resolve inconclusive findings
Bladder tumor	– Different morphologic appearance – Arises from the bladder
Prostatic utricle cyst	– Midline cystic lesion, located posterior and superior to the verumontanum, confined to the prostate or extends posteriorly beyond the prostate

Tips and Pitfalls

BPH may be mistaken for prostate cancer.

Selected References

Nicolas V et al. Prostata. In: Freyschmidt J, Nicolas V, Heywang-Köbrunner SH (eds). Handbuch diagnostische Radiologie. Heidelberg: Springer; 2004

Definition

Acute or chronic inflammation of the prostate • Chronic prostatitis is often abacterial • Typically caused by *Ureaplasma urealyticum*.

- **Epidemiology**
  Does not occur before puberty • Incidence increases with age • Usually an incidental finding in patients undergoing prostate biopsy for PSA elevation • Often occurs in association with UTI • Urinary tuberculosis involving the prostate in rare cases.

Imaging Signs

- **Modality of choice**
  Microbiological testing • Transrectal ultrasound.
- **Routine diagnostic workup**
  Microbiological testing of prostatic secretions or last sample of urine obtained in 3-glass test • Tender prostate on rectal examination • Possible transrectal ultrasound.
- **Transrectal ultrasound findings**
  Ultrasound is performed using a 7.5 MHz endoprobe • Good delineation of the prostate and seminal vesicles • Hypoechoic areas and liquefactions in the prostate.
- **MRI**
  MRI is not indicated in patients with clinically suspected prostatitis • Hypointense areas on T2-weighted images (as with prostate cancer) • Hypointense areas tend to be more inhomogeneous and sectorlike with the base directed toward the capsule • MR spectroscopy provides no additional information for clearly differentiating prostatitis and prostate cancer.

Clinical Aspects

- **Typical presentation**
  Acute prostatitis is common in men with lower UTI—dysuria, frequency, prostate tender on palpation • Chronic prostatitis is usually asymptomatic.
- **Treatment options**
  Specific antibiotic treatment.
- **Course and prognosis**
  Rapid resolution of the symptoms of acute prostatitis under antibiotic treatment • Several weeks of antibiotic treatment followed by PSA level determination in patients with elevated PSA before treatment • Prostate biopsy in case of persistent PSA elevation.
- **What does the clinician want to know?**
  Presence of complications such as liquefaction • Exclusion of prostate cancer.

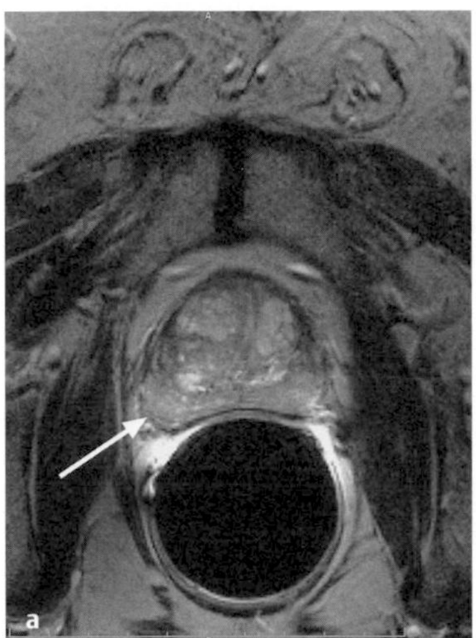

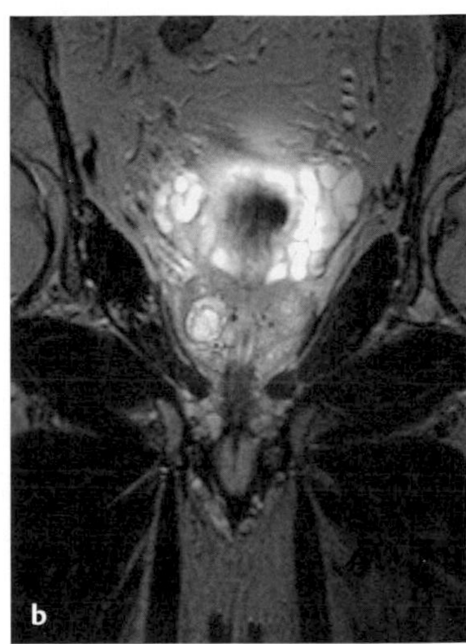

Fig. 3.19 a, b Prostatitis. Axial (**a**) and coronal (**b**) T2-weighted MR images. Hypointensity in the peripheral zone (arrow).

Differential Diagnosis

Prostatic hemorrhage	– Low signal intensity on T1-weighted images
Prostate cancer	– Signal reduction tends to be more homogeneous but reliable differentiation is not possible
Fibrosis	– History: after irradiation or hormone replacement therapy

Tips and Pitfalls

Imaging provides only little information in prostatitis because most findings are nonspecific • Wait at least 6 weeks before performing MRI after prostate biopsy (hemorrhage).

Selected References

Beyersdorff D, Hamm B. MRT zur Problemlösung beim Nachweis des Prostatakarzinoms. Röfo 2005; 177: 788–795

Nickel JC Classification and diagnosis of prostatitis: a gold standard? Andrologia 2003; 35: 160–167

Shukla-Dave A et al. Chronic prostatitis: MR imaging and ^{1}H MR spectroscopic imaging findings—initial observations. Radiology 2004; 231: 717–724

Definition

Adenocarcinoma is the most common malignant tumor of the prostate • Typically arises in the peripheral zone • Prostate cancer screening starting at age 50—PSA test and digital rectal examination.

- **Epidemiology**
  Incidence increases with age • Most common malignancy and second most common cause of cancer death in men • Estimated incidence of prostate cancer in the USA in 2006: 234 460 cases.
- **Staging**
  T1: Tumor identified by prostate biopsy.
  T2a: Tumor involves less than half of one lobe.
  T2b: Tumor involves more than half of one lobe.
  T2c: Tumor involves both lobes.
  T3a: Tumor extends into periprostatic fat.
  T3b: Tumor invades seminal vesicles.
  T4: Tumor invades adjacent structures—bladder, rectum, or striated pelvic floor muscles.
  N1: A minimal axial diameter over 10 mm is suggestive of lymph node metastasis.

Imaging Signs

- **Modality of choice**
  Transrectal ultrasound.
- **Routine diagnostic workup**
  - *Transrectal ultrasound with prostate biopsy:* Routine systematic biopsy (at least six specimens).
  - *Nuclear bone scan:* Screening for bone metastases; metastatic spread to the bones is unlikely up to a PSA of 10 ng/mL; areas of increased uptake are subsequently examined by radiography; CT to resolve inconclusive findings; high prevalence of osteoplastic bone metastases.
  - *Abdominal CT scan:* Lymph nodes.
  - *Chest radiograph.*
  - *MRI:* Indications—men with raised PSA levels but initially negative biopsy, staging of proven prostate cancer, hematospermia, and inconclusive findings on transrectal ultrasound or palpation.
- **Transrectal ultrasound findings**
  Ultrasound using a 7.5 MHz endoprobe • Good delineation of the prostate and seminal vesicles • Most prostate tumors are identified as hypoechoic focal lesions • Overall sensitivity and specificity are low • Therefore systematic prostate biopsy is required.
- **MRI findings**
  MRI performed with a combined endorectal body phased-array coil • Angulated axial and coronal T2-weighted TSE sequences and axial T1-weighted sequences • Slice thickness: 3 mm • Additional axial PD-weighted sequence up to the

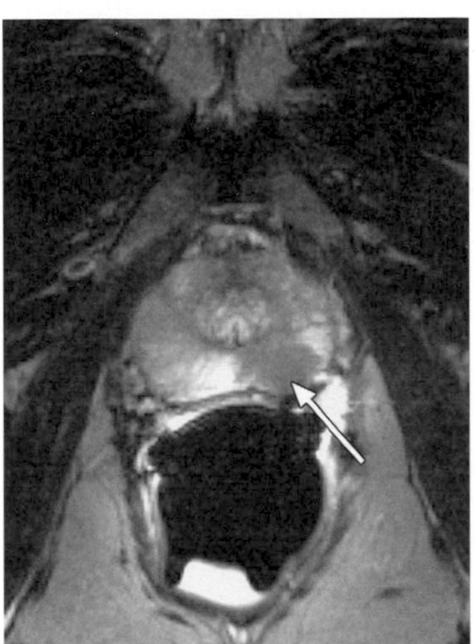

Fig. 3.20 Prostate cancer without extracapsular extension (T2b). Axial T2-weighted MR image with good visualization of the zonal anatomy. Hypointense tumor in the hyperintense peripheral zone.

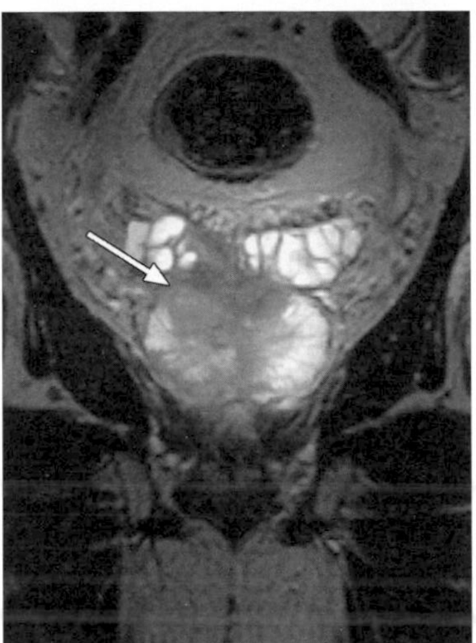

Fig. 3.21 Prostate cancer infiltrating the seminal vesicles (T3b). Coronal T2-weighted MR image. Hypointense area located centrally in the otherwise hyperintense seminal vesicles.

aortic bifurcation for lymph node evaluation • Good visualization of prostate zonal anatomy, the capsule, and adjacent structures such as the seminal vesicles and pelvic floor • T2-weighted sequences typically depict tumors as hypointense areas in the otherwise hyperintense peripheral zone.

Clinical Aspects

- **Typical presentation**
  Asymptomatic for a long time • Only larger tumors in the peripheral zone can be palpated • Urinary retention and obstruction as late complications • Worsening general condition in patients with metastatic prostate cancer.
- **Treatment options**
  Depend on the tumor stage • *Curative:* Radical prostatectomy, radiotherapy • *Palliative:* Hormone therapy, chemotherapy.
- **Course and prognosis**
  Prostate cancer typically grows slowly • Men with tumors that can be treated curatively have the best prognosis • *Therapeutic complications:* Impotence, urinary incontinence, voiding dysfunction.
- **What does the clinician want to know?**
  Location and extent of suspicious areas in the prostate before biopsy • Tumor extent and lymph node enlargement for therapeutic decision making.

Differential Diagnosis

BPH	– Transitional zone – Bulbous – Cannot always be differentiated by ultrasound
Prostatic hemorrhage	– High signal intensity on T1-weighted images
Prostatitis	– Typically more inhomogeneous signal reduction
Fibrosis	– History: after irradiation or hormone replacement therapy
Calcifications	– Acoustic shadowing on ultrasound – Signal voids on T1-weighted and T2-weighted images

Tips and Pitfalls

Wait at least 6 weeks before performing MRI after prostate biopsy (hemorrhage) • Do not use CT for prostate imaging.

Selected References

Beyersdorff D, Hamm B. MRT zur Problemlösung beim Nachweis des Prostatakarzinoms. Röfo 2005; 177: 788–795

Müller-Lisse UG, Scherr M. H1-MR-Spektroskopie der Prostata: Ein Überblick. Radiologe 2003; 43: 481–488

Pelzer A et al. Prostate cancer detection in men with prostate specific antigen 4 to 10 ng/ml using a combined approach of contrast enhanced color Doppler targeted and systematic biopsy. J Urol 2005; 173: 1926–1929

Definition

The formation of abnormal fibrous tissue in the two erectile bodies of the penis because of longstanding circulatory insufficiency.

- **Etiology**
  Arterial or venous cause (thrombosis, priapism, trauma) • Irreversible fibrous damage of the corpora cavernosa, resulting in complete loss of erectile function.

Imaging Signs

- **Modality of choice**
  MRI.
- **Pathognomonic findings**
  Reduced signal intensity of the corpora cavernosa on T2-weighted images • No contrast enhancement.
- **MRI findings**
  Marked and nearly homogeneous reduction of the normally high signal intensity of the corpora cavernosa (comparison with corpus spongiosum) on T2-weighted images • Moderate, homogeneous signal reduction of the corpora on unenhanced T1-weighted images • Markedly reduced contrast enhancement of the corpora cavernosa.

Clinical Aspects

- **Typical presentation**
  Erectile dysfunction.
- **Treatment options**
  Penile prosthesis.
- **What does the clinician want to know?**
  Diagnosis and exclusion of other, potentially curable conditions (e.g., acute thrombosis).

Differential Diagnosis

Acute corpus cavernosal thrombosis	– High signal intensity on unenhanced T1-weighted images in most cases (but varies with thrombus age) – Mass effect on the contralateral corpus cavernosum may occasionally be seen
Penile fracture	– Discontinuity of the tunica albuginea – Hematoma – Subacute soft tissue edema

Selected References

Horger DC et al. Partial segmental thrombosis of corpus cavernosum: case report and review of world literature. Urology 2005; 66: 194

Pretorius ES et al. MR imaging of the penis. Radiographics 2001; 21: S283–S299

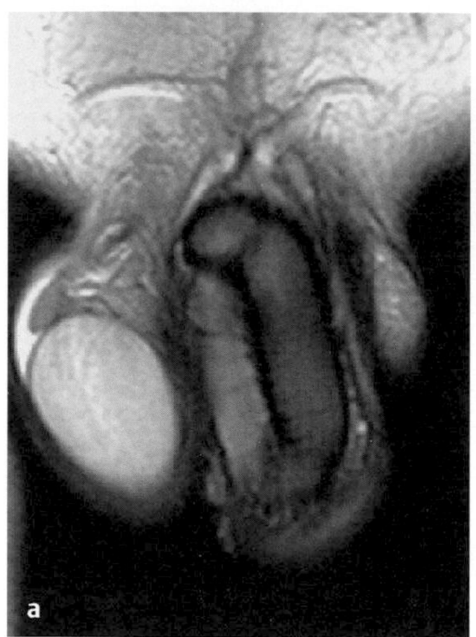

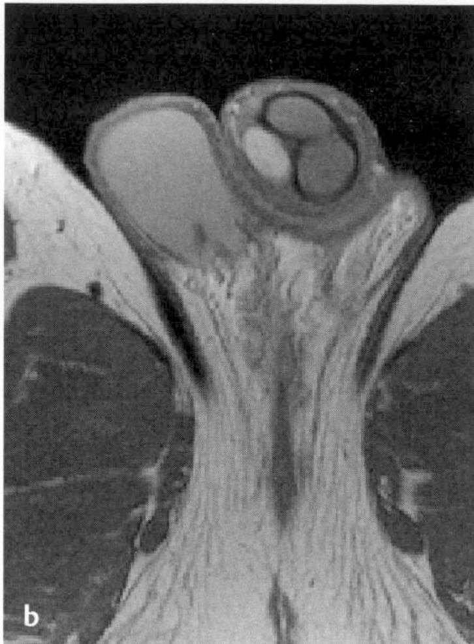

Fig. 3.22 a, b Fibrosis of the corpora cavernosa. MR images.

a Coronal T2-weighted TSE image. Note the difference between the homogeneous, hypointense fibrous corpus cavernosum and the normal hyperintense corpus spongiosum.

b Axial T1-weighted TSE image after contrast administration. No enhancement of the corpora cavernosa while the corpus spongiosum is enhanced (kindly provided by Dr. R. Dominik, Berlin).

Definition

A connective tissue disorder of the penis characterized by focal thickening of the tunica albuginea and intercavernosal septum (fibrous plaques) • *Synonyms:* Fibrous cavernositis and plastic induration of the penis.

- **Epidemiology**
  Peak incidence: Fourth to sixth decades of life • Association with other connective tissue disorders (especially Dupuytren contracture).
- **Etiology**
  Not definitely established: autoimmune etiology or trauma (microtrauma) • Characterized by initial acute inflammation with subsequent growth of fibrous plaques • Calcifications are very common • Plaques may lead to dorsal curvature of the penis.

Imaging Signs

- **Modality of choice**
  MRI • ultrasound mainly for follow-up.
- **Pathognomonic findings**
  Circumscribed inflammatory plaques of the tunica albuginea.
- **MRI findings**
  Plaques are hyperintense compared with normal tunica albuginea on T1- and T2-weighted images • Typically in the dorsal aspect of the penis • Signal voids indicate calcifications • Acute inflammation is associated with contrast enhancement of the plaques and possibly perifocal enhancement of the corpus cavernosum.
- **Ultrasound findings**
  Focal, hyperechoic thickening of the tunica albuginea • Posterior acoustic shadowing indicates calcifications.
- **Conventional radiograph (soft-beam technique)**
  Only if no other imaging modality is available • Demonstrates calcifications.

Clinical Aspects

- **Typical presentation**
  Pain during erection in the acute phase • Varying degrees of penile deformity • Erectile dysfunction.
- **Treatment options**
  Medical treatment (anti-inflammatory, immunosuppressive) • Surgical resection of plaques • Penile prosthesis when all other treatment options fail.
- **Course and prognosis**
  Spontaneous regression in 30–50% of patients • Men with chronic recurrent disease have an unfavorable prognosis.
- **What does the clinician want to know?**
  Extent of inflammatory process and response to treatment • Typically a clinical diagnosis (palpation, history, autophotography).

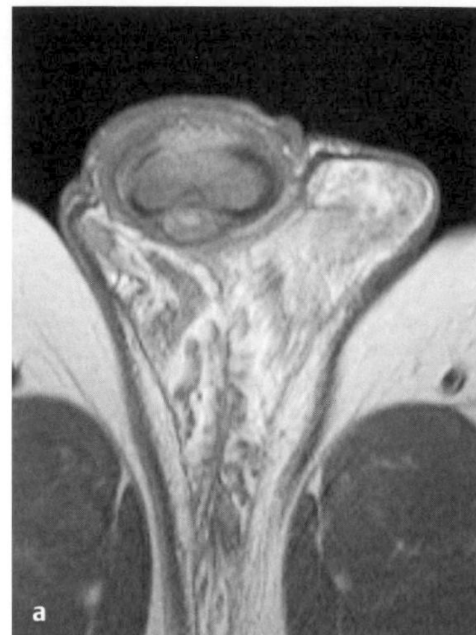

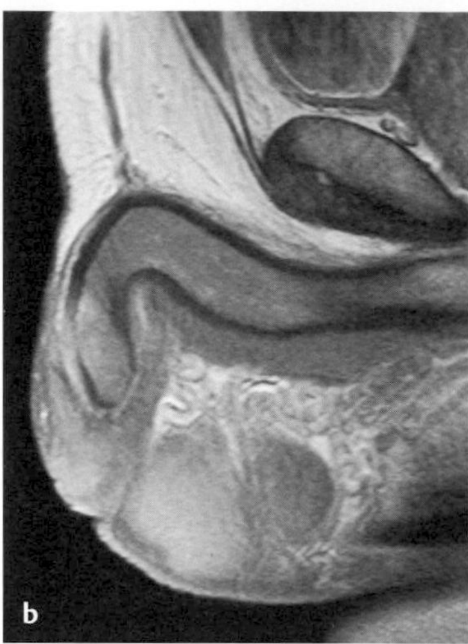

Fig. 3.23 a, b Peyronie disease. Plaque in typical location in the dorsal aspect of the penis. Axial (**a**) and sagittal (**b**) T1-weighted TSE MR images after contrast administration. Marked enhancement and focal thickening of the tunica albuginea. The enhancement of the plaque and surrounding corpus cavernosum indicates acute inflammation.

Differential Diagnosis

Scar formation after fracture	– Circular, nonfocal thickening of the tunica albuginea – No contrast enhancement – History

Tips and Pitfalls

MRI should ideally be done with a small surface coil to ensure adequate image quality • Fixation of the penis is necessary to prevent motion artifacts.

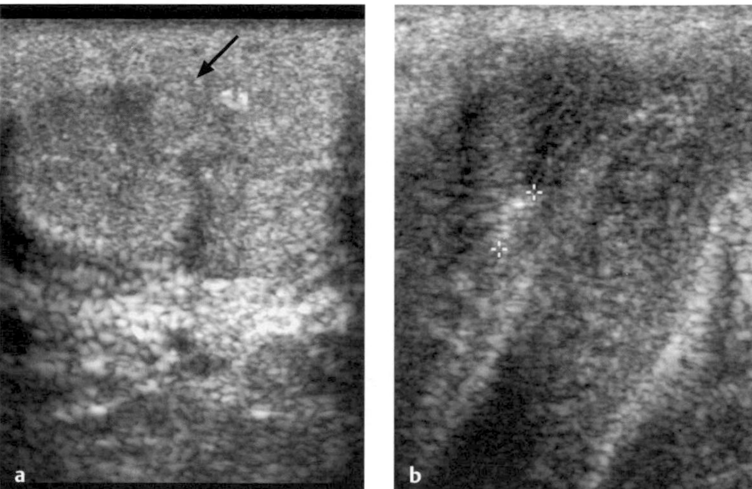

Fig. 3.24 a, b Peyronie disease. Plaque in the dorsal aspect of the penis. Transverse (**a**) and sagittal (**b**) ultrasound scans. The plaque extends into the intercavernosal septum (**a**). The otherwise hypoechoic tunica albuginea is hyperechoic in the vicinity of the plaque. Circumscribed area of increased echogenicity in the plaque represents calcification (**b**).

Selected References

Andresen R et al. Imaging modalities in Peyronie's disease. Eur Urol 1998; 34: 128–135

Fornara P, Gerbershagen HP. Ultrasound in patients affected with Peyronie's disease. World J Urol 2004; 22: 365–367

Hauck EW et al. Diagnostic value of magnetic resonance imaging in Peyronie's disease—a comparison both with palpation and ultrasound in the evaluation of plaque formation. Eur Radiol 2003; 43: 293–300

Definition

- **Epidemiology**
  Penile cancer and metastasis to the penis are the most common penile malignancies • Sarcoma and urothelial carcinoma of the male urethra are rare • *Peak incidence:* Fifth to seventh decades of life • Circumcised men have a lower risk of penile cancer.
- **Etiology**
  Squamous cell carcinoma: Association with HPV 16 and 18 • Most commonly located in the glans • *Metastasis:* Typically from a primary tumor in the urogenital tract (prostate, urothelial cancer).
- **Staging (according to Jackson)**
  - *Stage I:* Confined to the glans or prepuce.
  - *Stage II:* Involves the penile shaft (corpus cavernosum).
  - *Stage III:* Inguinal lymph node metastases.
  - *Stage IV:* Pelvic lymph node metastases.

Imaging Signs

- **Modality of choice**
  MRI.
- **MRI findings**
  Lesion of low signal intensity compared with the corpus cavernosum on T1- and T2-weighted images • Penile cancer is inhomogeneous • Metastasis is typically homogeneous • Less marked contrast enhancement than the corpus cavernosum.
- **Ultrasound findings**
  Hyperechoic lesion • Moderately vascularized.

Clinical Aspects

- **Typical presentation**
  Palpable swelling • (Malignant) priapism.
- **Treatment options**
  Radical surgical resection—(partial) penectomy.
- **Course and prognosis**
  Five-year survival rate of over 80% in patients with stage I penile cancer • Less than 20% for stage II or higher.
- **What does the clinician want to know?**
  Staging: Involvement of the corpus cavernosum.

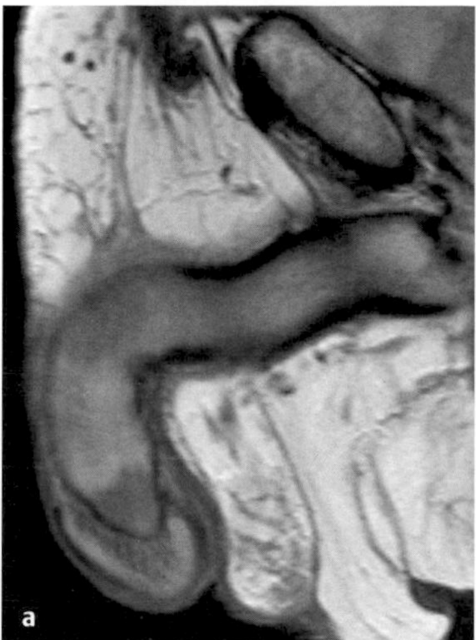

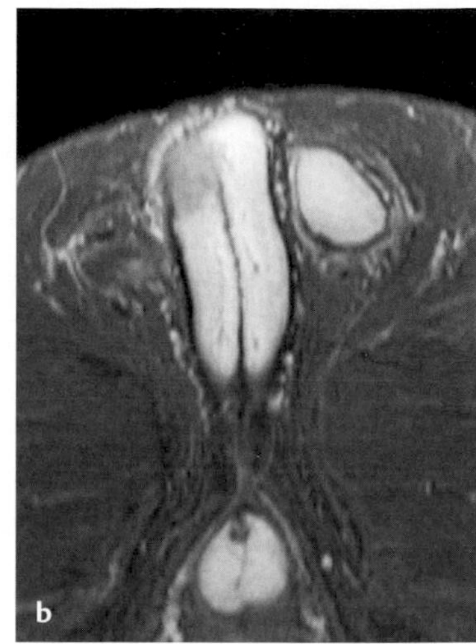

Fig. 3.25 a, b Two penile metastases from urothelial carcinoma; one in the dorsal aspect of the corpus cavernosum in the middle third of the penis, the other contiguous with the glans. Sagittal T1-weighted TSE (**a**) and axial T2-weighted IR (**b**) MR images depicting the metastases with lower signal intensity than the corpus cavernosum.

Differential Diagnosis

Partial thrombosis of the corpus cavernosum	– Often high signal intensity on T1-weighted images
Periurethral abscess	– Higher signal intensity than the corpus cavernosum on T2-weighted images – Rim enhancement
Cowper syringocele	– Higher signal intensity than the corpus spongiosum on T2-weighted images

Tips and Pitfalls

Carefully evaluate for inguinal lymph node metastases.

Selected References

Pretorius ES et al. MR imaging of the penis. Radiographics 2001; 21: S283–S299

Scardino E et al. Magnetic resonance imaging combined with artificial erection for local staging of penile cancer. Urology 2004; 63: 1158–1162

Singh AK et al. Imaging of penile neoplasms. Radiographics 2005; 25: 1629–1638

Definition

- **Anatomy**
  Uterus: 6–9 cm in length • Corpus-to-cervix ratio of 2:1 before menopause and 1:1 after menopause • Uterine corpus covered by peritoneum • Deflections of the peritoneum form the rectouterine pouch (pouch of Douglas, cul-de-sac) posteriorly and the vesicouterine pouch anteriorly • Position of the uterus changes with the degree of bladder and rectal filling (usually anteverted/anteflexed) • Uterine cervix projects into the vagina forming the lip or portio (ectocervix) and the fornix (vaginal vault), which flattens out anteriorly.
  Vagina: 8–10 cm long muscular tube • Lies within the paracolpium.
- **Layers**
  Cervix: Outer layer is the stroma consisting of connective tissue and isolated muscle fibers • Inner layer is the mucosa, which is thrown into deep irregular folds (palmate folds).
  Uterus: Outer layer is the myometrium • Inner layer is the endometrium • Appearance varies across the menstrual cycle • Endometrial layer is built up during the proliferative phase • Thickest in the mid-secretory phase.
  Parametrium: On both sides of the cervix • Fatty connective tissue containing the uterine venous plexus, uterine artery, and nerves.
  Paracolpium: Surrounds the vagina • Consists of fatty connective tissue and contains the paravaginal venous plexus • Contiguous with the parametrium above.

Imaging Signs

- **Modality of choice**
  MRI for evaluation of zonal anatomy.
- **MRI findings**
  Uterus: Three distinct zones on T2-weighted images: hyperintense endometrium, hypointense inner myometrium or junctional zone, and outer myometrium of intermediate signal intensity • Hyperintense mucus in the cavity on T2-weighted images • Intrauterine clots present in the secretory phase have high signal intensity on T1-weighted images • *Myometrium:* Increases in signal intensity and thickness in the first half of the cycle • Junctional zone: about 5 mm thick, hypointense, best delineated during the secretory phase • *Endometrium:* Thinnest just after menses, thickest in mid-cycle (10–14 mm) • Marked enhancement of endometrium and outer myometrium after contrast administration • *Postmenopausal uterus:* Thinner endometrium, no junctional zone, and lower myometrial signal intensity.
  Cervix: Three to four layers on T2-weighted images—very hyperintense mucus in the cervical canal (proliferative phase), hyperintense mucosa, hypointense inner stroma, hyperintense outer stroma • Parametria have heterogeneous, intermediate signal intensity on T2-weighted images.

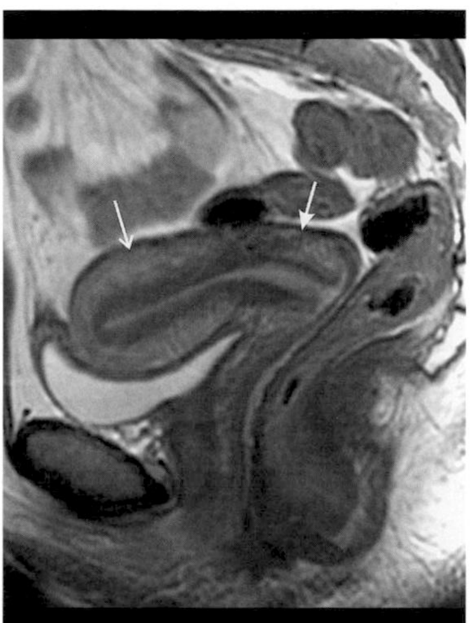

Fig. 4.1 Normal uterus of a 34-year-old woman during the first phase of the menstrual cycle. Sagittal T2-weighted MR image. Uterine zonal anatomy: outer uterine myometrium of intermediate signal intensity (open arrow), hypointense inner myometrium (junctional zone), and hyperintense endometrium. Cervix (filled arrow): moderately to slightly hyperintense stroma, and hyperintense mucosa and intraluminal mucus.

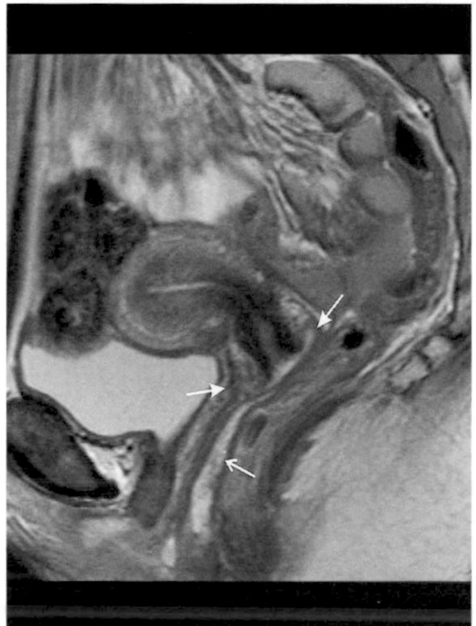

Fig. 4.2 Vagina of a 30-year-old woman during the first phase of the menstrual cycle. Sagittal T2-weighted MR image. Zonal anatomy: hyperintense paracolpium (open arrow), hypointense muscular layer, and innermost layer of hyperintense mucosa. Upper third of vagina: anterior and posterior fornix (filled arrows).

Vagina: Thin tube on T2-weighted images • W- or H-shaped in cross-section • Endoluminal mucus of very high signal intensity and hyperintense mucosa • Middle layer—the muscularis, which has lower signal intensity • Surrounded by hyperintense paracolpium.

Peritoneal fluid collection: Small amount of fluid in the pouch of Douglas is normal, especially around ovulation.

Tips and Pitfalls

The zonal anatomy is rather indistinct during the first half of the cycle • A small collection of fluid in the pouch of Douglas is normal and must not be mistaken for pathologic change.

Selected References

Hoad CL et al. Uterine tissue development in healthy women during the normal menstrual cycle and investigations with magnetic resonance imaging. Am J Obstet Gynecol 2005; 192: 648–654

Hricak H et al. Vagina: evaluation with MR imaging. Part I. Normal anatomy and congenital anomalies. Radiology 1988; 169: 169–174

Klüner C, Hamm B. Normal imaging findings of the uterus. In: Hamm B, Forstner R (eds). MRI and CT of the Female Pelvis. Heidelberg: Springer; 2006

Definition

- **Epidemiology**
  Uterine anomalies occur in 0.5% of women and vaginal anomalies in 0.025% • 39% are accounted for by bicornuate uterus and 34% by septate uterus • Associated malformations of the wolffian duct (kidneys, urinary tract) and urogenital sinus.
- **Etiology**
  American Fertility Society classification according to type of congenital defect:
  - *Dysgenesis:* Agenesis/hypogenesis of uterus or vagina, unicornuate uterus.
  - *Vertical fusion defects:* Cervical dysgenesis, transverse vaginal septa.
  - *Lateral fusion defects:* Didelphys, bicornuate, and septate uteri.

Imaging Signs

- **Modality of choice**
  MRI for morphologic assessment, classification, and surgical planning • Transvaginal ultrasound • Hysterosalpingography for assessing tubal patency.
- **MRI findings**
  Absence of uterus and upper vagina: Associated anomalies of the kidneys and urinary tract in 50% of cases • Condition also known as Mayer–Rokitansky–Küster–Hauser syndrome.
  Unicornuate uterus: Incomplete or absent development of one of the müllerian ducts • "Banana-shaped" single-horn uterus on one side • Rudimentary second horn with or without cavity may be present • Cavity of rudimentary horn may communicate with healthy cavity • Rudimentary horn may be distended by blood.
  Bicornuate uterus: Incomplete fusion of the müllerian ducts • Two separate uterine cavities • Divided by myometrial septum • Concave fundus • Greater distance between the two horns.
  - Arcuate uterus (mildest form of bicornuate uterus): Short septum (< 1 cm) extending only partially down the uterine cavity; flattened fundus.
  - Bicornuate unicollis uterus: Septum dividing uterus down to internal os.
  - Bicornuate bicollis uterus: Septum dividing uterus down to external os.
  - Didelphys uterus (most severe form of bicornuate uterus): Complete failure of müllerian duct fusion; two separate uterine bodies and cervices with vagina divided by septum; fundal concavity; increased intercornual distance.
  - Double uterus: Didelphys uterus without vaginal septum.

  Septate uterus: Normal müllerian duct fusion • Incomplete septal resorption • Slightly increased intercornual distance • Flattened/convex fundus.
  Vaginal septum: Horizontal fusion defect with formation of a vaginal septum • May lead to ipsilateral hematometrocolpos and ipsilateral hematosalpinx.

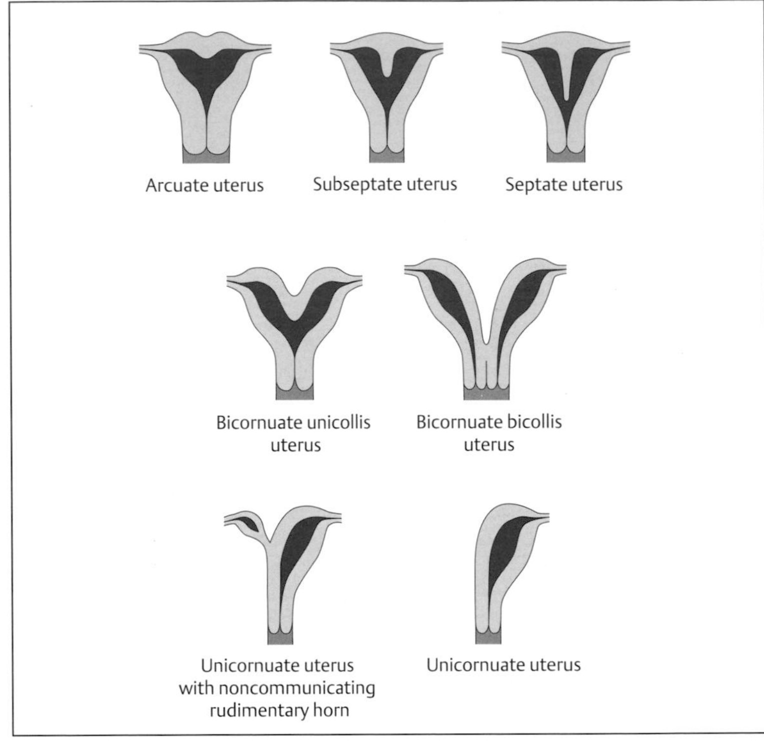

Fig. 4.3 Classification of uterine anomalies.

Clinical Aspects

- **Typical presentation**
  Primary amenorrhea • Dysmenorrhea • Infertility • Recurrent miscarriage • Complications during delivery.
- **Treatment options**
  Prompt repair of obstructive malformations • Bicornuate uterus can be left untreated in most cases • In women with symptoms, transabdominal septum resection and metroplasty for myometrial septum • Hysteroscopic resection of fibrous uterine septum • Vaginoplasty in vaginal atresia.
- **What does the clinician want to know?**
  Configuration of the uterine fundus • Intercornual distance • Intercornual angle • Presence of obstructions and blood • Uterine septa • Appearance of the vagina, ovaries, kidneys, and urinary tract • Presence of additional pelvic anomalies.

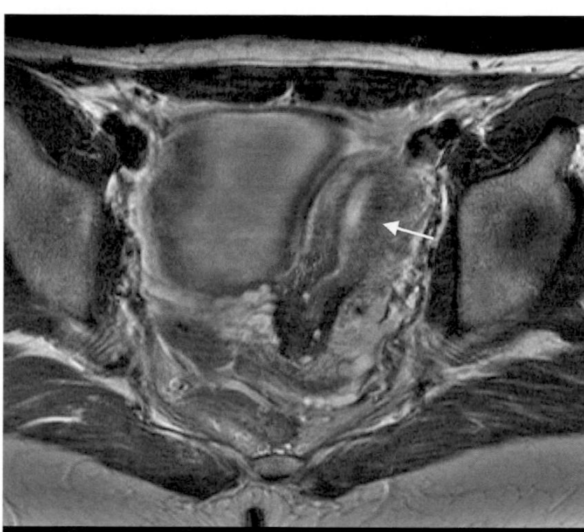

Fig. 4.4 Unicornuate uterus. Axial T2-weighted MR image. Single horn on the left side (arrow) and absent horn on the right.

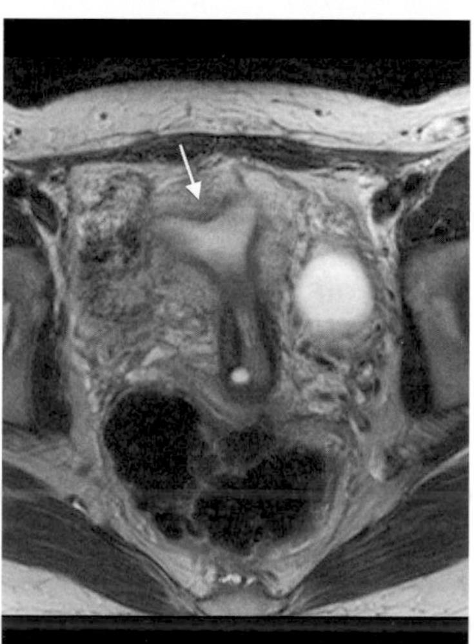

Fig. 4.5 Arcuate uterus. Axial T2-weighted MR image. Fundal concavity (arrow). Accessory finding: nabothian cyst.

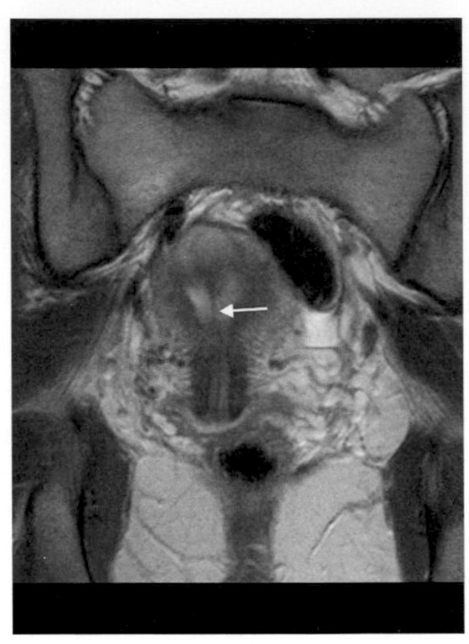

Fig. 4.6 Septate uterus. Angulated coronal T2-weighted MR image. The uterine cavity and cervical canal are divided by a fibrous septum (arrow).

Tips and Pitfalls

Also assess the kidneys and urinary tract for associated anomalies since they are common in women with uterine anomalies.

Selected References

Pellerito JS et al. Diagnosis of uterine anomalies: relative accuracy of MR imaging, endovaginal sonography, and hysterosalpingography. Radiology 1992; 183: 795–800

Roos J, Kubik-Huch R. Congenital malformations of the uterus. In Hamm B, Forstner R (eds). MRI and CT of the Female Pelvis. Heidelberg: Springer; 2006

Saleem SN et al. MR imaging diagnosis of uterovaginal anomalies: current state of the art. Radiographics 2003; 23: e13

Definition

- **Epidemiology**
  Nabothian cyst: Common finding in premenopausal women • *Bartholin cyst:* Common, occurs at any age • *Gartner duct cyst:* Less common.
- **Etiology**
  - *Nabothian cyst:* Retention cyst due to epithelial proliferation with localized overgrowth and obstruction of a cervical gland • *Cervical glands:* Develop as invaginations of the cervical mucosa (palmate folds).
  - *Gartner duct cyst:* Developmental remnants of the wolffian duct, usually in the lateral wall of the vagina or vulva.
  - *Bartholin cyst:* Obstruction of one of the paired greater vestibular glands (Bartholin glands) by an inflammatory process or trauma with retention of secretions.
  - *Bartholin abscess/empyema:* Chronic inflammation of a major vestibular gland, e.g., in gonorrhea • Typically unilateral.

Imaging Signs

- **Modality of choice**
  MRI.
- **MRI findings**
  - *Nabothian cyst:* Cervical cyst containing mucous secretions • High signal intensity on T2-weighed images • Typically a few millimeters in size, rarely several centimeters.
  - *Gartner duct cyst:* Thin-walled cystic lesion • High signal intensity on T1- and T2-weighted images • Ranges in size from a few millimeters to several centimeters
  - *Bartholin cyst:* Cyst near the vaginal opening • High signal intensity on T2-weighted images • Intermediate to high signal intensity on T1-weighted images depending on the protein contents • Up to 5 cm in size.
  - *Bartholin abscess/empyema:* Poorly defined, septated mass with a thickened wall and marked enhancement after contrast administration.

Clinical Aspects

- **Typical presentation**
  Typically an asymptomatic incidental finding • *Gartner duct cyst:* Usually small and asymptomatic, larger cyst can compress the vagina/urethra • *Bartholin abscess:* Tender on palpation.
- **Treatment options**
  Small cysts do not require treatment • *Bartholin abscess:* Incision and antibiotic treatment.
- **What does the clinician want to know?**
  Differentiation from lesions that require treatment.

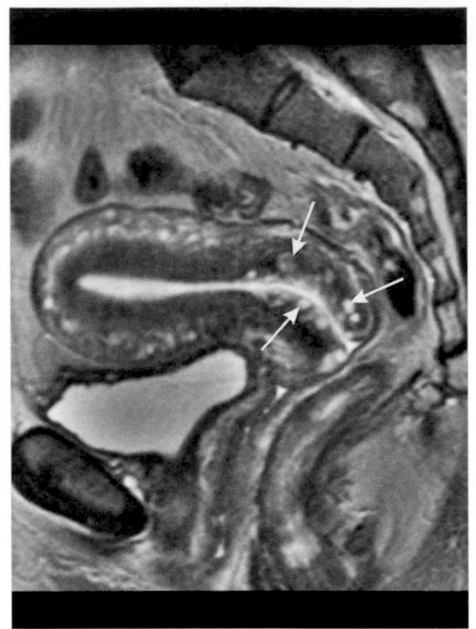

Fig. 4.7 Normal uterus with several nabothian cysts in the cervix (arrows). Sagittal T2-weighted MR image.

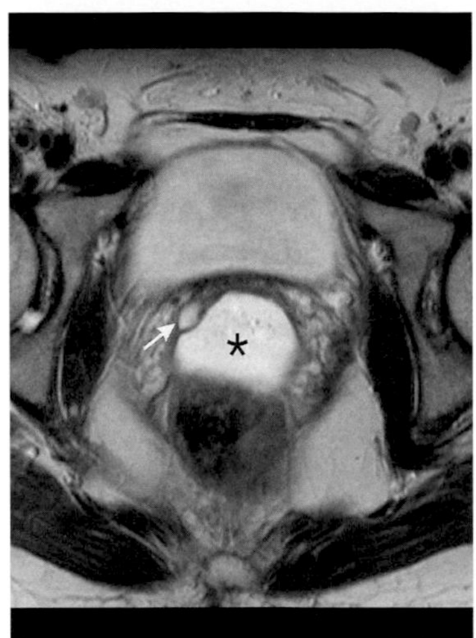

Fig. 4.8 Gartner duct cyst in the right anterior wall of the vagina (arrow). Axial T2-weighted MR image. Vagina filled with gel (asterisk).

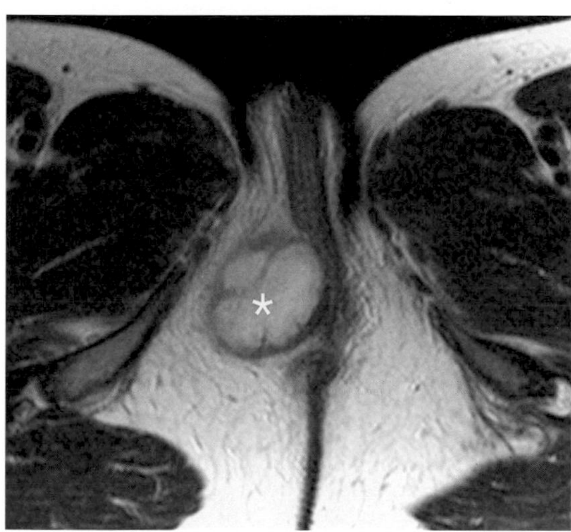

Fig. 4.9 Bartholin abscess (asterisk). Axial T2-weighted MR image. Inflammation is indicated by septation and thickening of the cyst wall.

Selected References

Hoad CL et al. Uterine tissue development in healthy women during the normal menstrual cycle and investigations with magnetic resonance imaging. Am J Obstet Gynecol 2005; 192: 648–654

Hricak H et al. Vagina: evaluation with MR imaging. Part I. Normal anatomy and congenital anomalies. Radiology 1988; 169: 169–174

Klüner C, Hamm B. Normal imaging findings of the uterus. In: Hamm B, Forstner R (eds). MRI and CT of the Female Pelvis. Heidelberg: Springer; 2006

Definition

Synonym: Fibroids.

▶ **Epidemiology**

Most common gynecologic neoplasm, accounting for over 30% of all uterine tumors • Typically occur before menopause • Often multiple • Ranging in size from a few millimeters to many centimeters • According to their location, leiomyomas are classified as intramural (55%), subserosal (35%), submucosal (5%), or cervical (5%).

▶ **Etiology**

Benign tumors composed of smooth muscle and fibrous connective tissue • Estrogen-dependent growth • Enlargement during pregnancy or oral contraceptive use • Degeneration of large fibroids and after menopause • *Sarcomatous transformation:* Most leiomyosarcomas arise independently of leiomyomas.

Imaging Signs

▶ **Modality of choice**

Ultrasound • MRI.

▶ **Ultrasound findings**

Well-circumscribed, homogeneous, hypoechoic mass • Hyperechoic areas indicate degeneration • Calcifications are identified by posterior shadowing • Anechoic areas represent liquid necrosis.

▶ **MRI findings**

Rounded tumor with well-circumscribed margins • Homogeneous, low to intermediate signal intensity on T2-weighted images • *Hyaline/myxoid degeneration:* Hyperintense areas on T2-weighted images and hypointense areas on T2-weighted images • *Cystic degeneration:* Hyperintensities on T2-weighted images • *Hemorrhagic/red degeneration:* Hyperintense rim on T1-weighted images and variable signal on T2-weighted images • *Calcifications:* Low signal intensity on T2-weighted images • *Necrosis:* Low signal intensity on T2-weighted images; liquid necrosis—high signal intensity on T2-weighted images and variable signal on T1-weighted images • *Pseudocapsule:* Hyperintense rim on T2-weighted images (compressed surrounding tissue, edema, dilated veins or lymphatic vessels) • Subserosal fibroids may become pedunculated and mimic ovarian tumors • Submucosal fibroids elevate the endometrium or may prolapse into the uterine cavity or even the cervix or vagina if they are pedunculated • Contrast administration is rarely necessary • More marked enhancement than the myometrium with higher signal intensity on T1-weighted images • Heterogeneous enhancement in case of degeneration (cysts, necrosis, calcifications) • Follow-up after uterine artery embolization (UAE)—reduced enhancement.

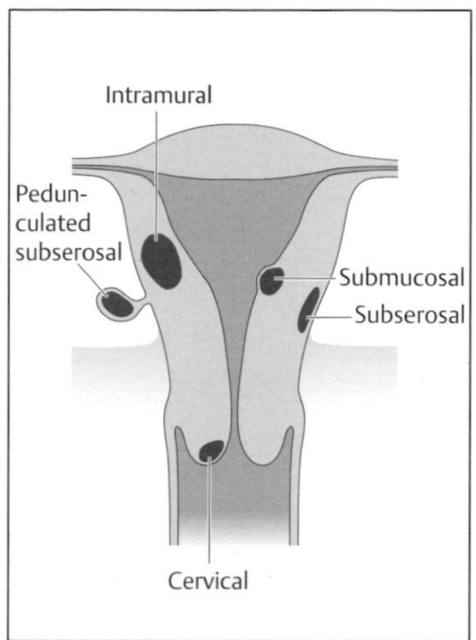

Fig. 4.10 Classification of uterine leiomyomas by location.

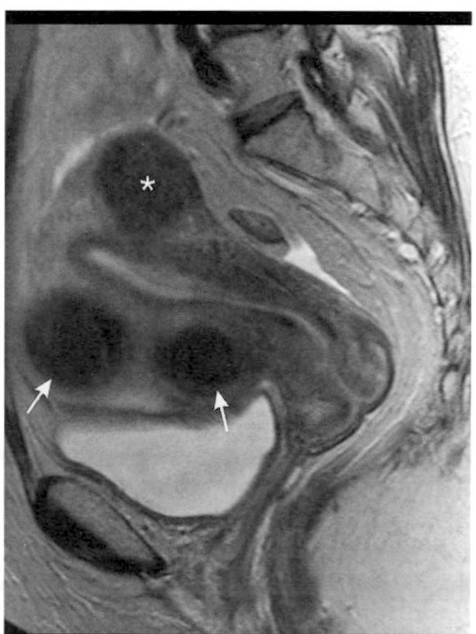

Fig. 4.11 Sagittal T2-weighted MR image. Two intramural leiomyomas (arrows) and one subserosal leiomyoma (asterisk).

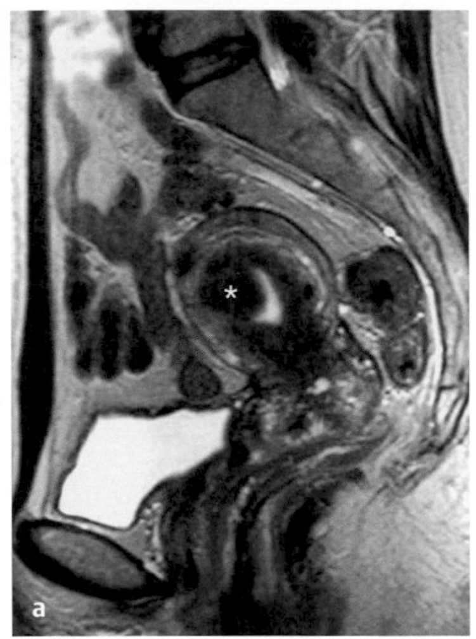

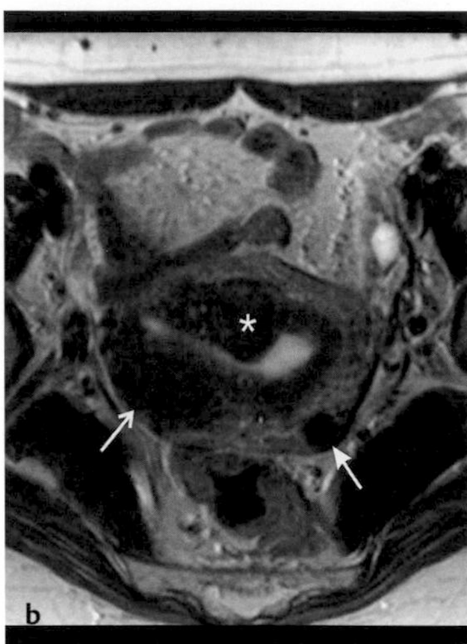

Fig. 4.12 a, b Sagittal (**a**) and axial (**b**) T2-weighted MR images. Submucosal leiomyoma (asterisk) protruding into the uterine cavity and a second, small leiomyoma (**b**, filled arrow) in the posterior wall of the uterus. Focal adenomyosis (open arrow) in the right posterior wall.

Clinical Aspects

- **Typical presentation**
  Asymptomatic (50–80%, intramural fibroids) • Dysmenorrhea • Menorrhagia, which may result in anemia • Infertility • Early abortion • Complications during delivery • *Large fibroids:* May compress adjacent organs (incontinence, obstipation), palpable pelvic mass, abdominal pain (degeneration) • *Subserosal fibroids:* Torsion with painful infarction.
- **Treatment options**
  Treatment is indicated for symptomatic fibroids and fibroids that enlarge after menopause • *Medical treatment:* GnRH analogue, gestagen • UAE • *Surgical options:* Enucleation (hysteroscopic, laparoscopic), hysterectomy.
- **What does the clinician want to know?**
  Number, size, and location of fibroids • Planning of UAE or surgery • Outcome of UAE or response to medical treatment.

Differential Diagnosis

Endometrial polyp, endometrial cancer	– Higher signal intensity than submucosal fibroid
Adenomyosis	– Originates in the junctional zone (inner myometrium) – Ill-defined – Less pronounced mass effect – Small foci of high signal intensity
Focal myometrial contractions	– Will resolve on subsequent imaging because contractions are transient – Ill-defined – No mass effect – Contiguous with the junctional zone
Ovarian fibroma	– No pedicle arising from the uterus
Uterine leiomyosarcoma	– Rapid growth (no reliable criterion)

Tips and Pitfalls

Care must be taken not to mistake focal adenomyosis for leiomyoma.

Selected References

Kröncke TJ. Benign uterine lesions. In: Hamm B, Forstner R (eds). MRI and CT of the Female Pelvis. Heidelberg: Springer, 2006

Murase E. Uterine leiomyomas: histopathologic features, MR imaging findings, differential diagnosis, and treatment. Radiographics 1999; 19: 1179–1197

Definition

- **Epidemiology**
  Affects about 25% of women • More common in multiparous women • Symptoms before menopause.
- **Etiology**
  Ectopic endometrial glands and stroma (basal endometrium) within the myometrium (junctional zone) accompanied by smooth muscle hyperplasia • Only little affected by cyclical hormonal changes • Associated with tamoxifen therapy • Often occurs together with uterine fibroids.

Imaging Signs

- **Modality of choice**
  Transvaginal ultrasound • MRI.
- **Ultrasound findings**
  Ill-defined, heterogeneous areas of low signal intensity within the myometrium • Myometrial cysts • Asymmetrically enlarged or globular uterus • Focal adenomyosis may be difficult to distinguish from leiomyoma.
- **MRI findings**
  Widening of the hypointense junctional zone (to at least 12 mm) on T2-weighted images • Often small foci of high signal intensity on T2-weighted images (ectopic endometrial tissue and dilated endometrial cysts) • *Focal adenomyosis:* Irregular and poorly defined mass causing localized thickening of the junctional zone • *Diffuse adenomyosis:* Changes throughout the uterus, which is often enlarged • Individual lesions are more conspicuous and resemble fibroids under GnRH analogue treatment • Contrast administration provides no additional information in most cases because enhancement is similar to that of normal myometrium.
  Rare forms:
  - Adenomyoma: Very well-defined focal adenomyosis • Punctate foci of high signal intensity may be seen.
  - Polypoid adenomyoma/adenomyomatous polyp: Adenomyoma characterized by polypoid protrusion into the uterine cavity.

Clinical Aspects

- **Typical presentation**
  Often asymptomatic • *Nonspecific symptoms:* Dysmenorrhea, menorrhagia • Uterine enlargement.
- **Treatment options**
  Treatment required only in symptomatic adenomyosis • Initial attempts with nonsteroidal anti-inflammatory drugs, danazol, GnRH • Hysterectomy (most common form of treatment) • Endometrial ablation • *New alternative approach:* Arterial embolization.

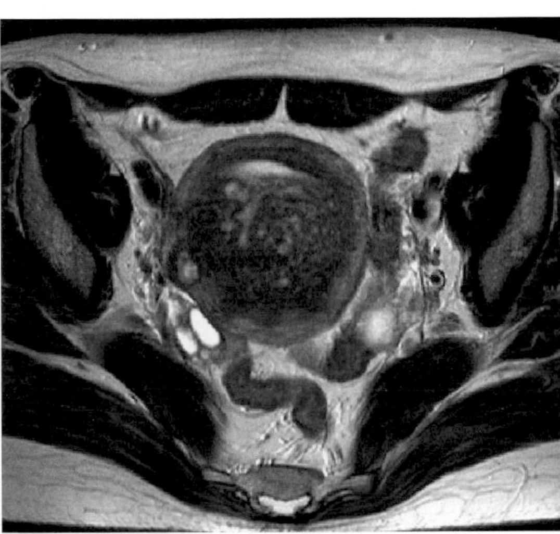

Fig. 4.13 Adenomyosis of the posterior uterine wall. Axial T2-weighted MR image. Small foci of high signal intensity in the thickened junctional zone.

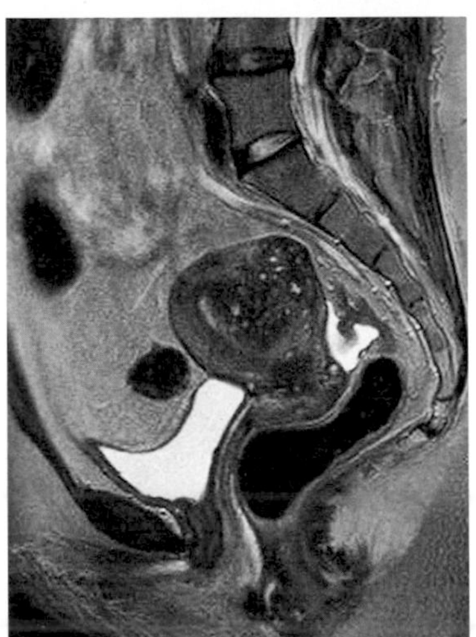

Fig. 4.14 Adenomyosis of the posterior uterine wall. Sagittal T2-weighted MR image. Typical small foci of high signal intensity.

► **What does the clinician want to know?**
Extent • Location • Differentiation from leiomyomas (different treatment) • Demonstration of adenomyosis in patients presenting with fertility problems.

Differential Diagnosis

Physiologic thickening of the junctional zone	– No hyperintense foci – Usually no thicker than 8 mm
Focal myometrial contractions	– Localized thickening of the junctional zone on T2-weighted images – Typically less than 12 mm – Transient—from minutes to a few hours; can be distinguished by resolution on subsequent imaging
Leiomyoma	– More rounded and better-defined tumor with a mass effect

Tips and Pitfalls

Correct differentiation of focal adenomyosis and leiomyoma is critical.

Selected References

Hamm B, Forstner R (eds). MRI and CT of the Female Pelvis. Heidelberg: Springer; 2006
Mark AS. Adenomyosis and leiomyoma: differential diagnosis with MR imaging. Radiology 1987; 163: 527–529
Tamai K. MR-imaging findings of adenomyosis: correlation with histopathologic features and diagnostic pitfalls. Radiographics 2005; 25: 21–40
Togashi K. Adenomyosis: diagnosis with MR imaging. Radiology 1988; 166: 111–114

Definition

- **Epidemiology**
  Affect about 10% of women • Multiple polyps in 20% of cases • Often develop around menopause.
- **Etiology**
  Benign, pedunculated focal mass of hyperplastic basal endometrium • Consists of glands, stroma, and vessels • Typically arises in the area of the fundus or tubal angles • Association with tamoxifen • Frequently found in association with leiomyoma and endometrial cancer • *Adenomyomatous polyp:* Contains muscle cells • Malignant transformation is rare (less than 1%).

Imaging Signs

- **Modality of choice**
  Ultrasound, MRI for differential diagnosis.
- **Ultrasound findings**
  Thickened endometrium • Localized mass may be present in the uterine cavity • More conspicuous on sonohysterography.
- **MRI findings**
  Pedunculated mass in the uterus • Slightly hypointense and more heterogeneous relative to the endometrium • Uterine cavity distended to 0.5–3 cm • Central fibrosis with lower signal intensity on T2-weighted images and more marked contrast enhancement • Cystic inclusions may be present • Marked contrast enhancement comparable to that of endometrium • Pedunculated polyps are thus delineated against the nonenhancing mucus • Irregular endometrial–myometrial interface at the site of attachment.

Clinical Aspects

- **Typical presentation**
  Usually asymptomatic • *Nonspecific symptoms:* Irregular bleeding • Most common cause of postmenopausal bleeding • Infertility.
- **Treatment options**
  Diagnostic and therapeutic dilatation and curettage • Any thickening of the endometrium over 5 mm with postmenopausal bleeding requires workup.

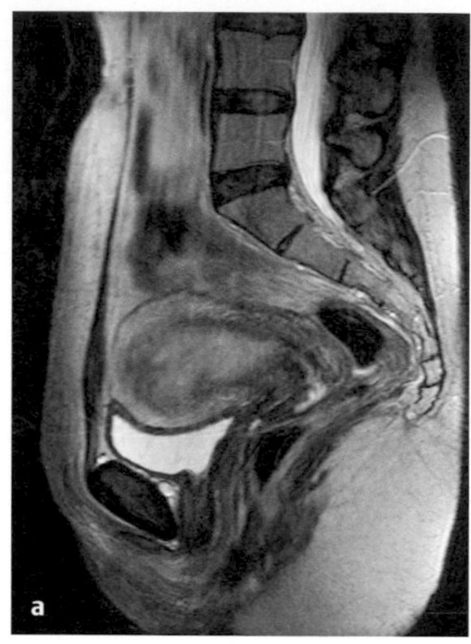

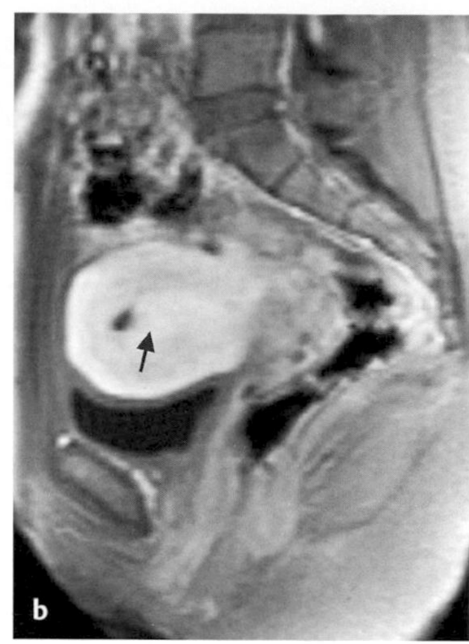

Fig. 4.15 a, b Endometrial polyp.

a Sagittal T2-weighted MR image. Thickening of the endometrium caused by a heterogeneous mass. The anterior interface of the junctional zone appears irregular.

b Sagittal T1-weighted MR image after contrast administration. The enhancing polyp is delineated against the nonenhancing mucus. The pedicle (arrow) of the polyp attaches to the anterior uterine wall.

Differential Diagnosis

Endometrial carcinoma	– Infiltration and thinning of the myometrium – No central fibrosis – Less marked contrast enhancement – Heterogeneous enhancement if necrotic areas are present – Early endometrial carcinoma (stage I) cannot be reliably differentiated
Endometrial hyperplasia	– Uniform endometrial thickening – Homogeneous contrast enhancement – Cystic inclusions – No central fibrosis – Cannot be differentiated from an endometrial polyp unless the lesion is outlined by endometrial mucus
Submucosal leiomyoma	– Lower signal intensity on T2-weighted images – Contiguous with the myometrium – Less marked contrast enhancement
Retained uterine secretions	– No contrast enhancement

Tips and Pitfalls

Always obtain a contrast-enhanced MR scan • Since a definitive diagnosis of an endometrial polyp cannot be made, the radiologic report should always discuss the likelihood of endometrial cancer and endometrial hyperplasia in the differential diagnosis.

Selected References

Chaudhry S et al. Benign and malignant diseases of the endometrium. Topics Magn Reson Imaging 2003; 14: 339–358

Grasel RP et al. Endometrial polyps: MR imaging features and distinction from endometrial carcinoma. Radiology 2000; 214: 47–52

Imaoka I et al. Abnormal uterine cavity: differential diagnosis with MR imaging. Magn Reson Imaging 1999; 17: 1445–1455

Nalaboff KM et al. Imaging the endometrium: disease and normal variants. Radiographics 2001; 21: 1409–1424

Takeuchi M et al. Pathologies of the uterine endometrial cavity: usual and unusual manifestations and pitfalls on magnetic resonance imaging. Eur Radiol 2005; 15: 2244–2255

Definition

- **Epidemiology**
  Affects about 10% of women in their reproductive years, typically between 30 and 45 years of age.
- **Etiology**
  Ectopic functional endometrial tissue outside the uterine cavity that responds to cyclic hormonal stimulation • Rarely there may be malignant transformation (2.5%) • Sites of involvement—ovaries (most common), peritoneum.
  Deep endometriosis:
  - Posterior: Pouch of Douglas • Parametria • Cervix • Vagina • Fallopian tubes • Intestine • Ureters.
  - Anterior: Bladder • Abdominal wall (rare, scars, umbilicus).

  Extraperitoneal involvement: Lungs • CNS (very rare).

Imaging Signs

- **Modality of choice**
  Laparoscopy • Ultrasound • MRI.
- **Ultrasound findings**
  Ovarian endometriotic cysts: avascular masses with diffuse low-level internal echoes and hyperechoic wall foci • Bladder wall involvement—hypoechoic nodules • Ultrasound is limited in evaluating involvement of more posterior structures.
- **MRI findings**
  MRI enables good visualization of endometriotic cysts but will not always detect implants (and contrast administration may be required).
  Endometriotic cysts (chocolate cysts): Nodular masses • Several millimeters to centimeters in diameter • No contrast enhancement • High signal intensity on T1-weighted images, which persists on fat-saturated images (distinguishing endometriotic cysts from dermoids) • T2-weighted images—loss of signal within the lesion (shading); layering due to blood products of different ages and concentrations • Thin septa in large cysts • Organ displacement and distortion of normal anatomy due to adhesions • Hypointense fibrous capsule • *Fibrous implants (plaques):* Low signal intensity on T1- and T2-weighted images with punctate foci of high signal intensity, enhancement after contrast administration.
  Ovaries: Often multiple lesions • Bilateral in 50% of cases • More marked contrast enhancement of adjacent peritoneum • Adhesions can cause posterior displacement or join the ovaries ("kissing ovaries") • Small implants on the surface.
  Uterus/Parametria: Very often in the uterosacral ligament, pouch of Douglas, and posterior cervix (torus uterinus) • Often bilateral • May be stellate or arched in shape • Asymmetric enhancement • Vaginal, rectal, and rectosigmoid adhesions • Hydrosalpinx.
  Vagina: More common in the posterior wall • Elevation of the posterior vaginal fornix.
  Intestine: Typically involving the rectosigmoid colon, pouch of Douglas, and rectovaginal septum • Rarely in the ileum, appendix, or cecum • Nodular thicken-

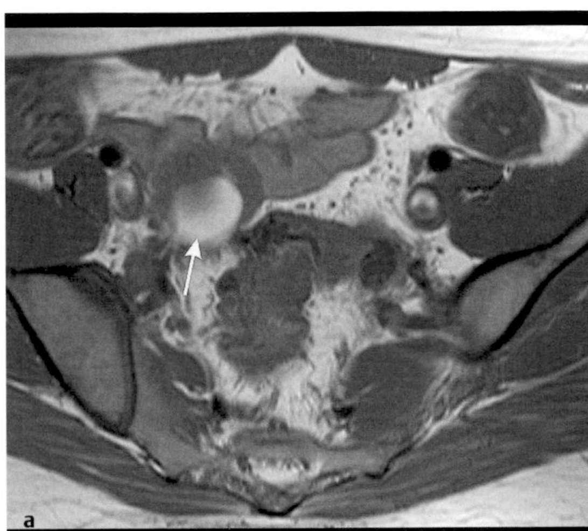

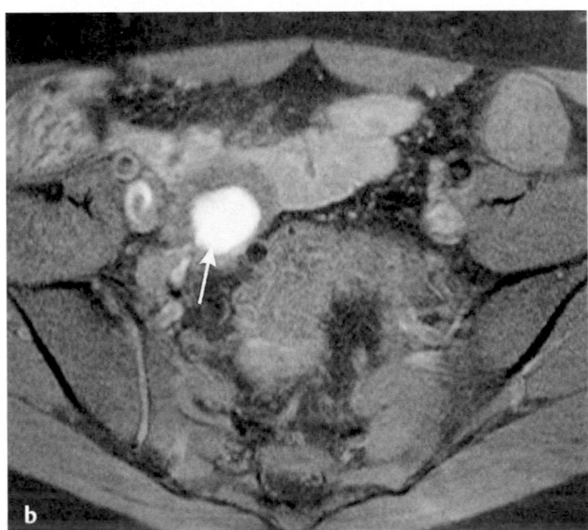

Fig. 4.16 a, b Endometriosis.
a Axial T1-weighted MR image. Endometriotic cyst (arrow) of the right ovary.
b Axial T1-weighted MR image with fat saturation. High signal intensity of the cyst contents (arrow) indicates presence of hemorrhage.

ing of the intestinal wall and adjacent peritoneum • Mucosa is spared • Adhesions to the uterus • Strictures • Deformities.
Bladder: Typically involving the dome or posterior wall (vesicouterine pouch, vesicovaginal septum, detrusor muscle) • Wall thickening with hemorrhagic cysts • Increased contrast enhancement.
Ureters: Compression and obstruction • Hypointense extensions due to retractions.

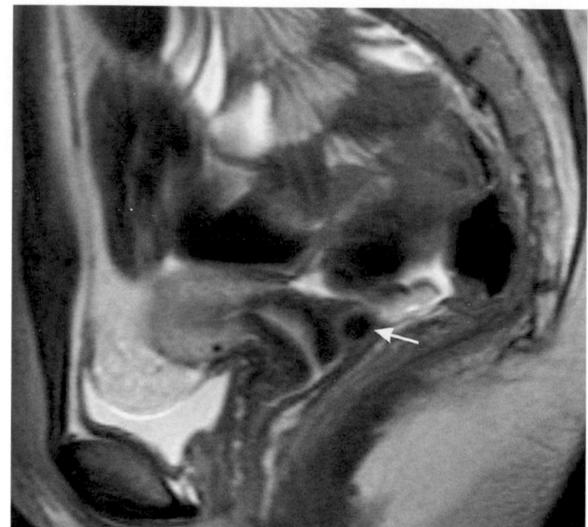

Fig. 4.17 Endometriosis. Sagittal T2-weighted MR image showing hypointense, rounded endometriotic cyst (arrow) in the pouch of Douglas.

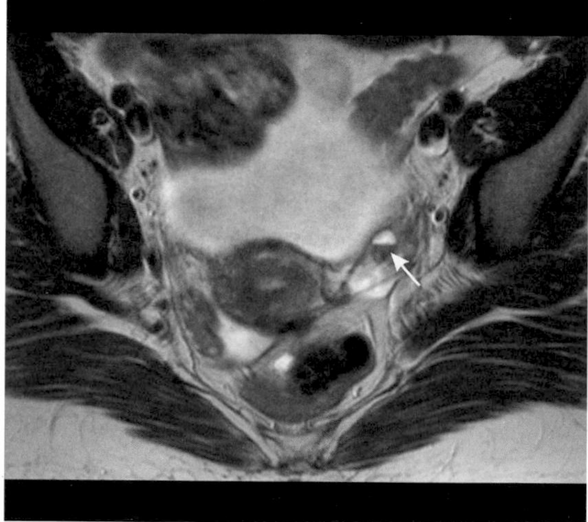

Fig. 4.18 Endometriosis. Axial T2-weighted MR image. Rounded lesion in the dome of the bladder (arrow) with layering indicating hemorrhage.

Peritoneum: Plaque • Hypointense stellate configurations may be present • Multilocular fluid collections.
Abdominal wall: Hyperintense foci on T1-weighted images.
Malignant transformation: Malignant mucinous tumor of the ovaries—contrast enhancement of the cyst.

Clinical Aspects

- **Typical presentation**
  Dysmenorrhea, typically 1–3 days before menstruation • Pelvic pain • Dyspareunia • Other manifestations according to site of involvement—enlarged uterus, infertility, tubal pregnancy, intestinal adhesions or bloody stools, cyclic pain and swelling of the abdominal wall • Improvement of symptoms after menopause.
- **Treatment options**
  Medical: Gestagen, GnRH agonist (danazol), GnRH analogue (goserelin) • Laparoscopic resection with hysterectomy and salpingo-oophorectomy in severe cases.
- **What does the clinician want to know?**
  Location • Presence of adhesions • Organ involvement (in particular intestine and bladder) for surgical planning.

Differential Diagnosis

Ovarian cysts	– Fluid contents with low signal intensity on T1-weighted images and high signal intensity on T2-weighted images – Functional cysts decrease in size – Smooth, thin capsule; no septa
Dermoid, teratoma	– Demonstration of fatty components: high signal intensity on T1- and T2-weighted images, low signal on fat-saturated T1-weighted images
Ovarian neoplasia	– Solid mass with or without cystic components, enhancement of solid parts, hyperintense areas on T1-weighted images
Protruding subserosal leiomyoma	– Contiguous with the uterus, pedunculated – Low signal intensity on T1-weighted images – Increase in signal intensity after contrast administration

Tips and Pitfalls

Perform MRI in the second half of the menstrual cycle • Obtain a fat-saturated T1-weighted sequence to differentiate blood (endometriosis) and fat (teratoma).

Selected References

Kinkel K, Chardonnens D. Endometriosis. In Hamm B, Forstner R (eds). MRI and CT of the Female Pelvis. Heidelberg: Springer; 2006

Kinkel K. Diagnosis of endometriosis with imaging: a review. Eur Radiol 2006; 16: 285–298

Woodward PJ et al. Endometriosis: radiologic-pathologic correlation. Radiographics 2001; 21: 193–216

Definition

Synonym: Corpus cancer.

- **Epidemiology**
  Most common female genital malignancy • Develops after menopause • *Peak incidence:* 55–70 years.
- **Etiology**
  Risk factors: Chronic estrogen exposure—unopposed postmenopausal estrogen replacement therapy or ovarian dysfunction (polycystic ovary syndrome, estrogen-producing ovarian tumor) • Long-term tamoxifen treatment for breast cancer (estrogenlike endometrial effects) • Obesity and diabetes mellitus • Women with hereditary nonpolyposis colorectal cancer (HNPCC) have an increased risk and typically develop endometrial carcinoma before 50 years of age.
- **Histology**
  Over 95% are adenocarcinomas, among them 75% of the endometrioid type • Papillary serous, adenosquamous and clear cell histotypes have a poor prognosis but are rare • Uterine sarcoma accounts for 1–3%.

Imaging Signs

- **Modality of choice**
  Transvaginal ultrasound • Additional MRI for treatment planning, e.g., if the uterus is markedly enlarged or fixed, or if cervical, ovarian, and peritoneal involvement is suspected.
- **Ultrasound findings**
  Thick hyperechoic endometrium • Ill-defined • Large cysts • Distended endometrial cavity.
- **MRI findings**
  Endometrial thickening from a homogeneous or lobulated mass • High signal intensity on T2-weighted images • Less marked enhancement after contrast administration than in the myometrium.
  - *Stage IA:* Intact junctional zone with smooth endometrial-myometrial interface.
  - *Stage IB:* Invasion of less than half the myometrium.
  - *Stage IC:* Invasion of more than half the myometrium.
  - *Stage II:* Endocervical glandular involvement or cervical stromal invasion.
  - *Stage III:* Tumor invades serosa or adnexa, or vaginal metastasis.
  - *Stage IVA:* Invasion of bladder or rectal mucosa.
  - *Stage IVB:* Pelvic and/or paraaortic lymphadenopathy.

  Recurrent endometrial cancer: Typically involves vaginal vault or pelvic sidewall • Indicated by enhancement after contrast administration.

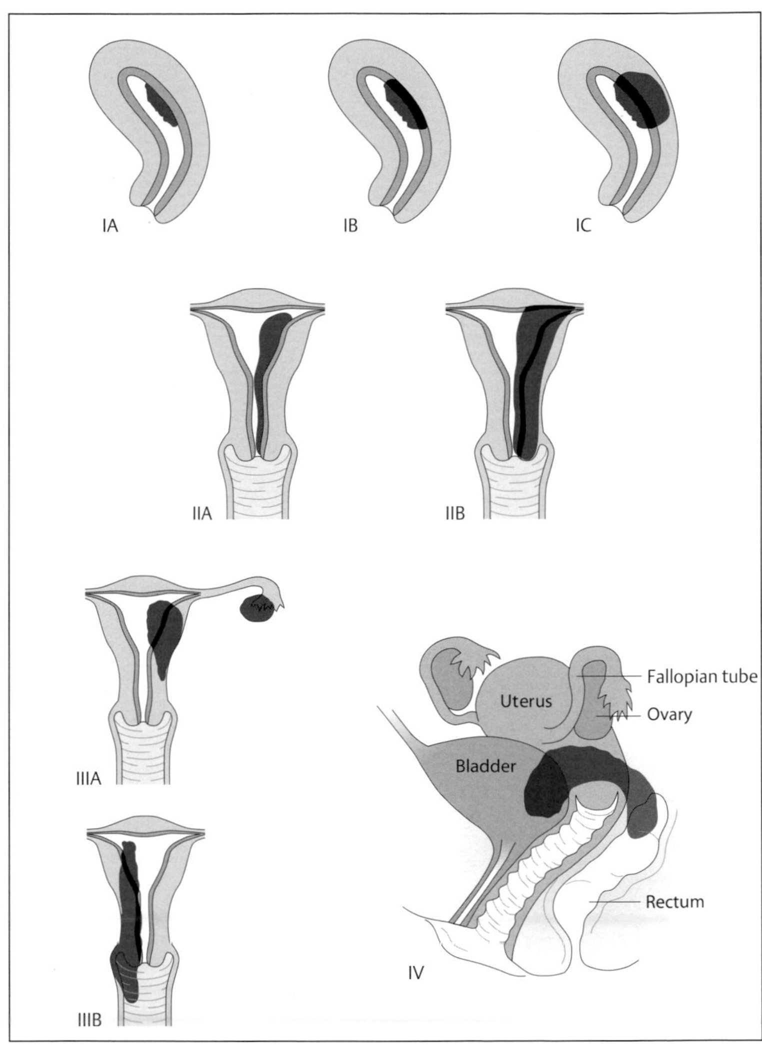

Fig. 4.19 FIGO and TNM stages of endometrial carcinoma.

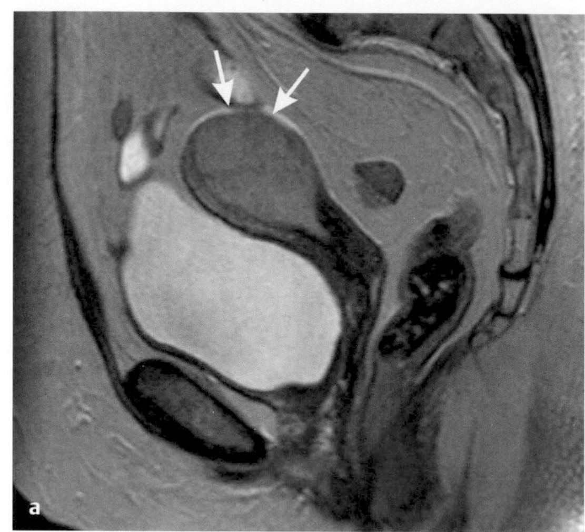

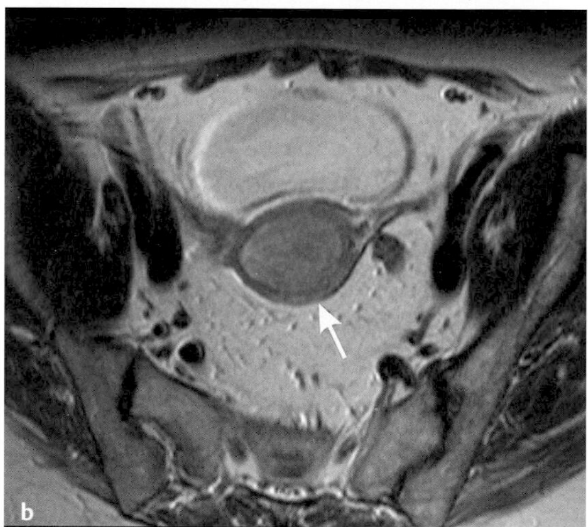

Fig. 4.20 a–c Endometrial carcinoma. Sagittal (**a**) and axial (**b**) T2-weighted MR images. Stage IC endometrial carcinoma. Large hyperintense mass in the uterine corpus invading the outer half of the myometrium (arrows). Less marked enhancement of the tumor compared with myometrium on contrast-enhanced T1-weighted MR image with fat saturation (**c**).

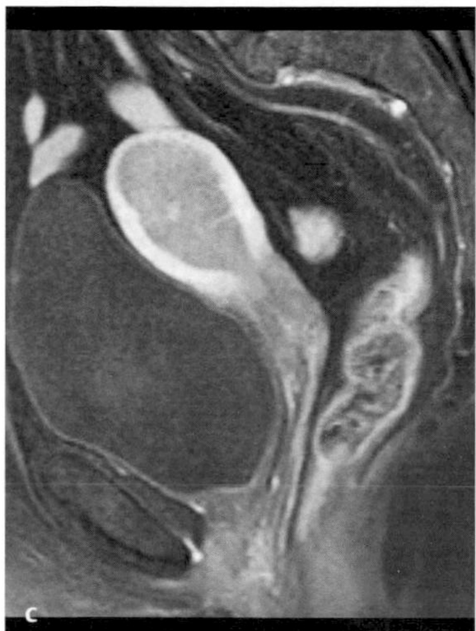

Clinical Aspects

- **Typical presentation**
  Presents early with postmenopausal bleeding and discharge.
- **Treatment options**
  Hysterectomy and possible bilateral salpingo-oophorectomy for stage IA/B disease with pelvic and paraaortic lymphadenectomy (stage IC) plus adjuvant radiotherapy as needed • Primary radiotherapy, adjuvant hormone therapy with progesterone, and chemotherapy in case of extrauterine tumor extension.
- **Course**
  Transserosal spread with direct invasion of adjacent organs and peritoneal seeding is rare • Late lymphatic spread to pelvic lymph nodes (internal, external, and common iliac and obturator nodes) • Spread to para-aortic lymph nodes via the tube, ovary, and ovarian suspensory ligament • Infiltration of inguinal nodes from the lower vagina or via the uterine appendages and round ligament • Hematogenous metastatic spread to the lungs, liver, and bones is rare.
- **Prognosis**
  Depends on tumor stage (FIGO), grading, histotype, and lymph node status • 5-year survival rate of 80% in stage I endometrial cancer, 5% in stage IV.
- **What does the clinician want to know?**
  Depth of myometrial invasion • Invasion of the cervix • Adnexal involvement • Presence of lymph node metastases.

Differential Diagnosis

Blood clot	– No contrast enhancement
Endometrial polyp	– Pedunculated – More marked contrast enhancement – No signs of malignant growth, no necrosis
Endometrial hyperplasia, normal endometrium	– Cannot be reliably differentiated from stage IA endometrial carcinoma – More marked contrast enhancement – No signs of malignant growth, no necrosis
Mixed müllerian tumor, endometrial stromal sarcoma	– Endometrial mass of high signal intensity – Cannot be differentiated from endometrial carcinoma on the basis of MR morphology

Tips and Pitfalls

Uterine zonal anatomy is less distinct in postmenopausal women due to regression of the junctional zone • Myometrial thinning in the presence of a large endometrial tumor or concomitant adenomyosis/leiomyoma may mimic myometrial infiltration • Prolapse of a tumor into the cervical canal may be difficult to distinguish from cervical invasion.

Selected References

Frei KA. Staging endometrial cancer: Role of magnetic resonance imaging. J Magn Reson Imaging 2001; 13: 850–855

Frei Bonel KA, Kinkel K. Endometrial Carcinoma. In: Hamm B, Forstner R (eds). MRI and CT of the female pelvis. Heidelberg: Springer; 2006

Hricak H et al. Endometrial cancer of the uterus. ACR Appropriateness Criteria. Radiology 19; 215 Suppl: 947–953

Kim S et al. Detection of deep myometrial invasion in endometrial carcinoma: Comparison of transvaginal ultrasound, CT and MRI. J Comput Assist Tomogr 1995; 19: 766–772

Sironi S. Myometrial invasion by endoemtrial carcinoma: assessment with plain and gadolinium enhanced MR-imaging. Radiology 1992; 185: 207–212

Definition

- **Epidemiology**
  Eighth most common malignancy in women; incidence has decreased in countries with screening programs • Second most common cause of cancer death in developing countries • Mean age at presentation is 52 years • Two peaks in incidence—at 35 and 70 years.
- **Etiology**
  Squamous cell carcinoma is the most common type (> 80%) • Arises in the transformation zone due to persistent infection with high-risk HPV. *Cofactors:* Sexual intercourse at a young age, multiple sexual partners, poor genital hygiene, frequent genital infections, immunocompromised state (e.g., HIV), smoking, vitamin deficiency • *Stepwise development:* Epithelial proliferation, dysplasia, precancerous states (CIN, SIL), carcinoma in situ, invasive carcinoma • 15% are adenocarcinomas.

Imaging Signs

- **Modality of choice**
  MRI for pretherapeutic staging and in patients with suspected recurrence.
- **MRI findings**
  Hyperintense cervical mass on T2-weighted images • Polypoid exophytic, diffusely infiltrating, or necrotic exulcerative growth • Infiltration of the hypointense cervical stroma.
  - *Stage IA:* Invasive cancer identified only microscopically • Not seen on MRI.
  - *Stage IB:* Cancer not extending beyond the uterus with intact stromal ring.
  - *Stage IIA:* Tumor involves the vagina but not its lower third.
  - *Stage IIB:* Parametrial invasion • Disruption of the cervical stroma • Mass in adjacent parametria.
  - *Stage IIIA:* Tumor involves the lower third of the vagina • Segmental high signal intensity in the otherwise hypointense vaginal wall.
  - *Stage IIIB:* Tumor extends to the pelvic sidewall or causes hydronephrosis.
  - *Stage IVA:* Tumor invades mucosa of the bladder or rectum • Segmental high signal intensity in the normally hypointense bladder or rectal wall.
  - *Stage IVB:* Tumor extends beyond the true pelvis or metastatic spread to distant organs.
  - *Metastatic spread:* Metastatic involvement of pelvic lymph nodes is the most important prognostic factor • Metastases of paraaortic nodes are classified as distant metastases • Late hematogenous spread to bones, lungs, peritoneum, and liver.

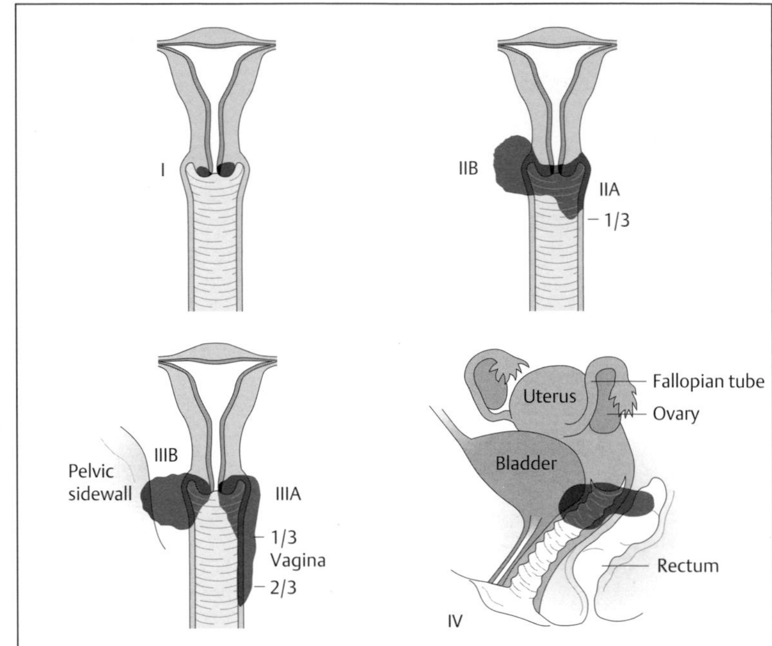

Fig. 4.21 FIGO and TNM stages of cervical cancer.

Clinical Aspects

- **Typical presentation**
  Early stages are asymptomatic • Detected at screening • Vaginal discharge and bleeding, pelvic pain, and painful intercourse in more advanced disease • Fatigue • Weight loss.
- **Treatment options**
  Depend on stage • *Surgery:* Radical hysterectomy and lymphadenectomy are usually performed for cervical cancer up to stage IIA • Primary, adjuvant, or neoadjuvant percutaneous radiotherapy or brachytherapy with simultaneous chemotherapy.
- **Prognosis**
  Prognostic factors: Tumor size, grade, local extent, lymph node status • 5-year survival rate of 88% in stage I, 73% in stage IIB, and 30% in case of pelvic organ involvement • Paraaortic lymph node metastases reduce survival by 50%.
- **What does the clinician want to know?**
  Tumor size • Tumor extent • Suspected parametrial invasion or involvement of pelvic organs • Pelvic lymph node status • Paraaortic nodal status in advanced disease.

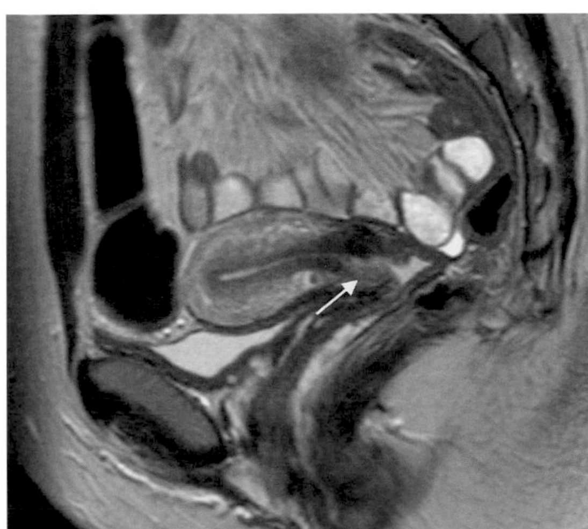

Fig. 4.22 Stage IB cervical cancer. Sagittal T2-weighted MR image. Cervical cancer (arrow) with anterior extension into the hypointense cervical stroma.

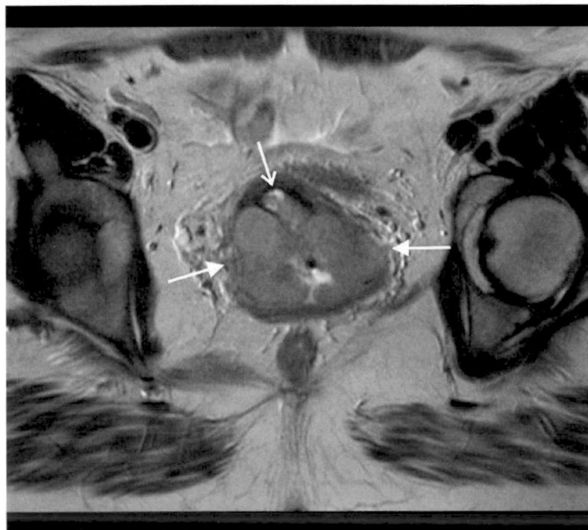

Fig. 4.23 Stage IIB cervical cancer. Axial T2-weighted MR image. Complete invasion of the cervical stroma from 3 o'clock to 10 o'clock and bilateral extension to the parametria (filled arrows). Cervical canal (open arrow).

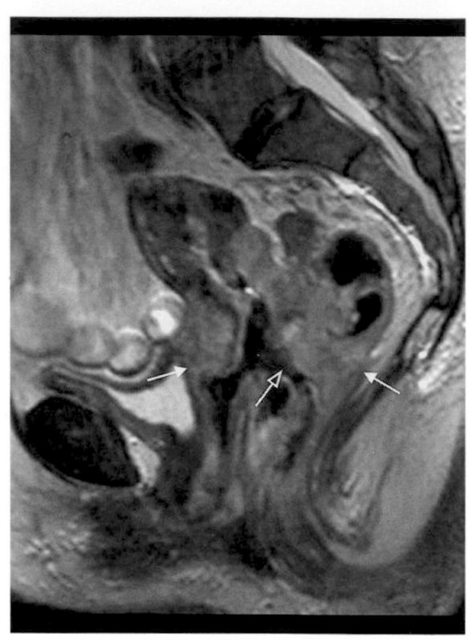

Fig. 4.24 Stage IVA cervical cancer. Sagittal T2-weighted MR image. Cervical cancer invading the vagina and rectum (filled arrows). A rectovaginal fistula is seen as a hypointense defect (empty arrow) within the tumor.

Differential Diagnosis

Cervicitis	– Superficial signal increase – No mass effect
Cervical metastasis	– Typically from endometrial cancer, less commonly from ovarian and breast cancer or melanoma

Tips and Pitfalls

Do not use CT for staging cervical cancer • Focal thickening of the cervical mucosa may mimic cervical cancer • Use MRI only for staging of histologically proven cancer • Always obtain angulated axial T2-weighted images • Perform contrast-enhanced study in patients with suspected fistula • Wait at least 6 months before performing follow-up MRI after surgery or radiotherapy. Otherwise hyperintensities might be misinterpreted as recurrent tumor.

Selected References

Follen M et al. Imaging in cervical cancer. Cancer 2003; 98(9 Suppl): 2028–2038

Nicolet V et al. MR imaging of cervical carcinoma: A practical staging approach. Radiographics 2000; 20: 1539–1549

Okamoto Y et al. MR Imaging of the uterine cervix: Imaging-pathologic correlation. Radiographics 2003; 23: 425–445

Zaspel U, Hamm B. Cervical cancer. In: Hamm B, Forstner R (eds). MRI and CT of the Female Pelvis. Heidelberg: Springer; 2006

Definition

- **Epidemiology**
  Two percent of all malignancies of the female genital tract • 80% after age 60 • Metastatic disease to the vagina (80%) is much more common.
- **Etiology**
  Squamous cell carcinoma accounts for over 90% of primary vaginal malignancies • Primary carcinoma associated with vaginal intraepithelial neoplasia • Often induced by high-risk HPV and other risk factors—multiple sexual partners, immunosuppression, smoking • 4% are adenocarcinomas—in younger women frequently associated with in utero exposure to diethylstilbestrol • Sarcoma is rare—embryonal rhabdomyosarcoma (sarcoma botryoides) in infants • Vaginal metastases typically originate from malignant tumors of the uterus, vulva, ovaries, bladder, rectum, and colon.

Imaging Signs

- **Modality of choice**
  MRI for staging of histologically proven carcinoma of the vagina.
- **MRI findings**
  Hyperintense tumor in the hypointense muscular vaginal wall on T2-weighted images • Early signal increase on contrast-enhanced images • Perfusion defects indicate regressive changes in larger tumors • Continuous growth with posterior extension to the rectovaginal fascia and rectum, anterior extension into the urethra and bladder, lateral invasion of paravaginal tissues and pelvic wall, and inferior extension to the perineum and anus.
  - *Stage I:* Vaginal wall deformity but tumor confined to vagina.
  - *Stage II:* Vaginal wall irregularity • Tumor invades paravaginal tissues.
  - *Stage III:* Tumor extends to pelvic wall and pelvic floor • Segmental disruption of the hypointense muscle layer by hyperintense tumor on T2-weighted images.
  - *Stage IV:* Tumor invades mucosa of the bladder and rectum • Extends beyond the true pelvis.

  T1-weighted sequence for nodal imaging: spread to inguinal lymph nodes from the lower vagina and to pelvic nodes (obturator, iliac, perirectal) from the upper two thirds • *Sarcoma botryoides:* Polypoid cystic tumor in the vagina.

Clinical Aspects

- **Typical presentation**
  Vaginal discharge • Spotting • Palpable firm nodular mass.
- **Treatment options**
  Stage I tumor: Partial or total vaginectomy with radical hysterectomy and inguinal/pelvic lymhadenectomy • *Tumor extending beyond the vagina:* Radiotherapy and exenteration • *Sarcoma botryoides:* Chemotherapy and surgery.

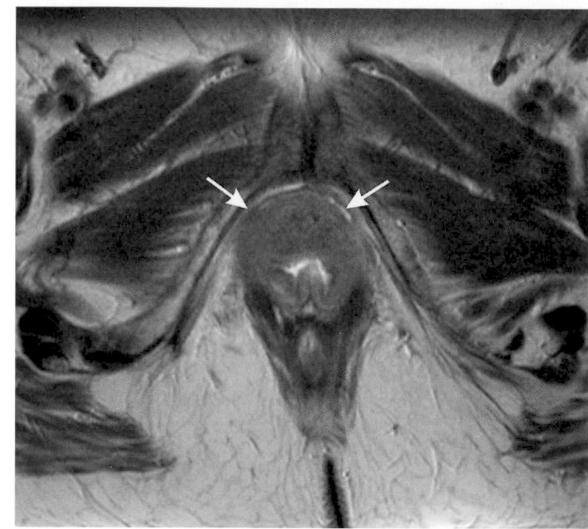

Fig. 4.25 Vaginal cancer. Axial T2-weighted MR image. Stage II cancer of the lower vagina (arrows) extending beyond the vagina and encasing the urethra.

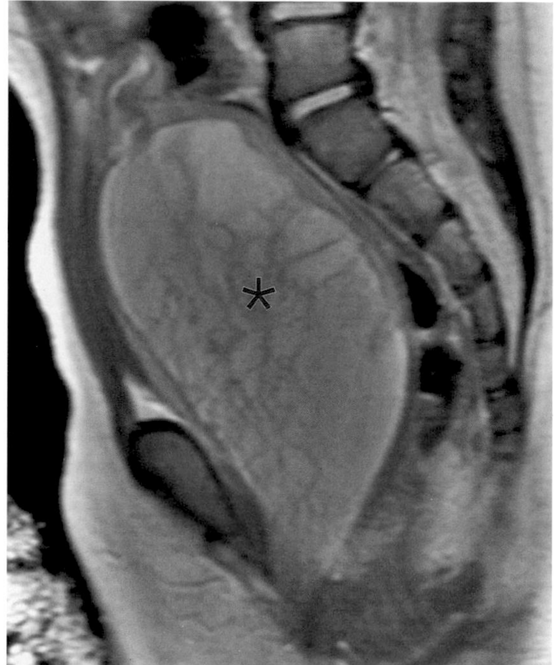

Fig. 4.26 Sarcoma botryoides in a 2-year-old girl. Sagittal T2-weighted MR image. Septated mass (asterisk) causing marked enlargement of the vagina.

- ▶ **Course**
  Direct local extension in the true pelvis • Lymphatic metastatic spread • Hematogenous metastatic spread occurs very late.
- ▶ **Prognosis**
  Depends on tumor stage, size, lymph node status, grade, and histotype • 10-year survival rate is 80% for stage I and 40% for stage III.
- ▶ **What does the clinician want to know?**
  Tumor size and spread in the true pelvis • Lymph node status.

Differential Diagnosis

Secondary vaginal malignancies	– History – Tumor usually originates in the organ with the largest tumor mass – Cannot be differentiated on the basis of their MR signal intensity characteristics, except for melanoma
Vaginitis, e.g., after brachytherapy	– Tends to cause circular, uniform thickening of the vaginal wall – Does not extend beyond the wall

Tips and Pitfalls

Very small vaginal carcinoma without invasion into the muscular layer cannot be differentiated from the hyperintense mucosa • Cancer difficult to distinguish from reactive inflammation or hemorrhage after biopsy • Contrast-enhanced T1-weighted sequence with fat saturation is helpful to differentiate introital tumor from the surrounding fat of the vulva.

Selected References

Chang YC. Vagina: evaluation with MR imaging. Part II. Neoplasms. Radiology 1988; 169: 175–179

Creasman WT. Vaginal cancers. Curr Opin Obstet Gynecol 2005; 17: 71–76

Hricak H. Vagina: evaluation with MR imaging. Part I. Normal anatomy and congenital anomalies. Radiology 1988; 169: 169–174

Siegelman ES. High-resolution MR imaging of the vagina. Radiographics 1998; 17: 1183–1203

Zaspel U, Hamm B. Vagina. In: Hamm B, Forstner R (eds). MRI and CT of the Female Pelvis. Heidelberg: Springer; 2006

Definition

- **Epidemiology**
  Five percent of all gynecologic tumors • *Peak incidence:* 60–70 years • 30% occur before menopause.
- **Etiology**
  90% squamous cell carcinomas • 10% basaliomas • Melanoma is rare • Adenocarcinoma arising in the vulvar glands is rare • *Predisposing factor:* HPV infection • *Precancerous state:* VIN.

Imaging Signs

- **Modality of choice**
  Inspection • MRI to resolve inconclusive findings and in patients with recurrent tumor.
- **MRI findings**
  Mass with intermediate signal intensity on T2-weighted images • Early lymphatic spread to ipsi- and contralateral inguinal and pelvic lymph nodes • Rarely there may be late hematogenous spread to the liver, lungs, and bones • Staging according to FIGO and TNM classification.
  - *Stage I:* Confined to the vulva or perineum, 2 cm or less in greatest dimension.
  - *Stage II:* Confined to the vulva or perineum, larger than 2 cm.
  - *Stage III:* Invasion of the lower urethra, vagina, or anus (seen on T2-weighted images as disruption of the hypointense wall by tumor of higher signal intensity).
  - *Stage IV:* Invasion of the upper urethra, bladder, rectum, or bony pelvis • Disruption of the hypointense muscle layer or bony cortex by hyperintense tumor on T2-weighted images.
  - *Inguinal and pelvic lymph node metastases:* Round, enlarged, absence of fatty hilum, necrosis.

  Recurrent vulvar cancer typically arises locally or from deep inguinal or femoral lymph nodes • High signal intensity on T2-weighted images • MRI not earlier than 6 months after the end of treatment to distinguish recurrence from inflammatory processes.

Clinical Aspects

- **Typical presentation**
  Induration and thickening of the vulva • Ulceration • Pruritus • Bleeding • Oozing • Pain.
- **Treatment options**
  Radical local excision or radical vulvectomy, usually with vulvar reconstruction • Inguinal lymph node dissection • Adjuvant radiotherapy as needed.
- **Prognosis**
  Depends on tumor size and depth of infiltration • 5-year-survival rate of 80% for cancer without involvement of inguinal lymph nodes, 40% for inguinal nodal involvement, and 20% for pelvic nodal involvement.

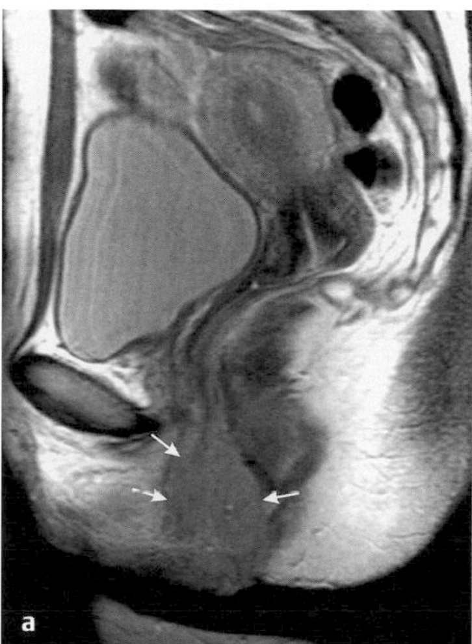

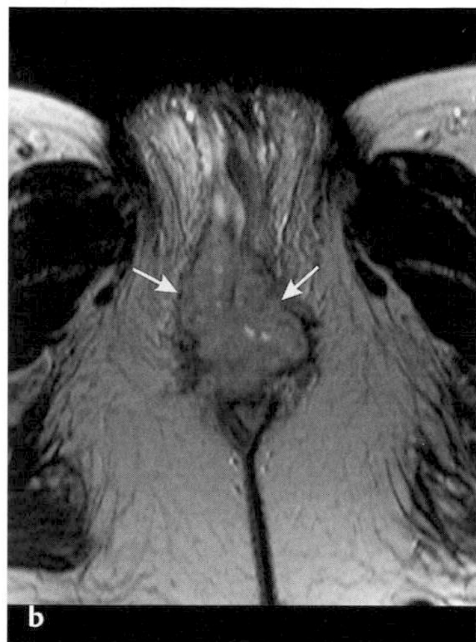

Fig. 4.27 a, b Vulvar carcinoma (arrows). Sagittal (**a**) and axial (**b**) T2-weighted MR images. Infiltration of the labia majora, external urethral orifice, and anal sphincter muscle.

▸ **What does the clinician want to know?**
Tumor spread: Involvement of the urethra, vagina, and rectum • Lymph node metastases.

Differential Diagnosis

Chronic vulvar inflammation	– Cannot be differentiated from superficial vulvar carcinoma
Bartholin cyst	– Thin-walled cyst not enhancing after contrast administration – Well-defined, no invasive growth

Tips and Pitfalls

Very small superficial vulvar carcinoma may be undetectable by MRI • Early infiltration of adjacent structures (clitoris, external urethral meatus, vaginal opening, anal sphincter) is difficult to distinguish from direct contact • Lymphadenopathy may also be due to inflammation of the genital organs.

Selected References

Hawnaur JM et al. Identification of inguinal lymph node metastases from vulval carcinoma by magnetic resonance imaging: an initial report. Clin Radiol 2002; 57: 995–1000

Sohaib SA et al. MR imaging of carcinoma of the vulva. Am J Roentgenol 2002; 178: 373–377

Definition

Abnormal descent of the pelvic floor and pelvic organs.

- **Epidemiology**
  History of several vaginal deliveries • Sixth and seventh decades of life.
- **Etiology**
  Weakness of the pelvic floor muscles, ligaments, and supporting structures • Descent of the uterus and vagina causes bulging of the anterior or posterior vaginal wall, which may result in the formation of a cystocele or rectocele • Often accompanied by enterocele (small intestine) and less commonly by sigmoidocele.

Imaging Signs

- **Modality of choice**
  MR defecography: Filling of the rectum (e.g., with ultrasound gel) and provocative maneuver (asking patient to strain to increase intraabdominal pressure) under "MR fluoroscopy".
- **Pathognomonic findings**
  Downward displacement of the bladder floor and cervix below the pubococcygeal line.
- **MRI findings**
  Provocation causes the uterus to protrude into the vagina with the cervix or bladder floor descending below the pubococcygeal line:
  - Mild: less than 3 cm.
  - Moderate: 3–6 cm.
  - Severe: over 6 cm.

  Anterior rectocele: Herniation greater than 2 cm anterior to a line extended up from the anal canal • Increased signal intensity of the levator ani muscle compared to the internal obturator muscle on T2-weighted images due to edema or higher fat content (atrophy) • Slackening of the levator ani muscle, which is usually straight (on transverse images).
- **Conventional defecography**
  Same findings as on MRI • Requires additional opacification of the vagina and bladder.

Clinical Aspects

- **Typical presentation**
  Stress urinary incontinence • Sensation of heaviness or pressure in the area of the vagina • Rectal incontinence.
- **Treatment options**
  Pelvic floor exercises • Pessary • Sling procedures • Vaginoplasty.

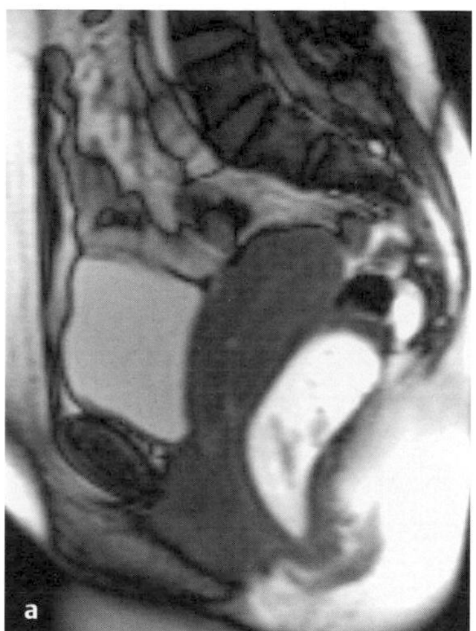

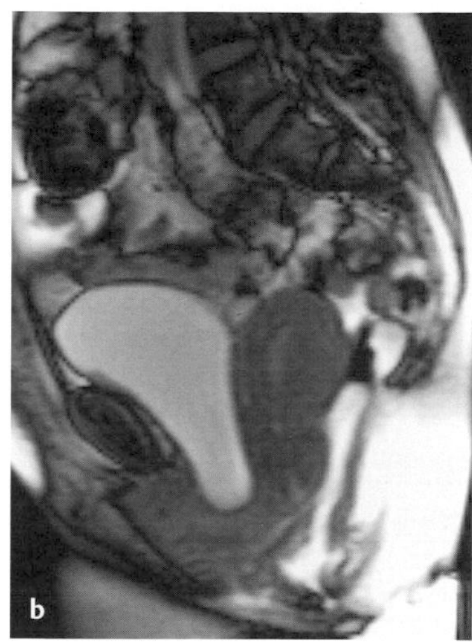

Fig. 4.28 a, b Pelvic organ prolapse. MR defecography. Filling of the rectum with ultrasound gel. Sagittal bSSFP sequence at rest (**a**) and during defecation (**b**). There is abnormal descent of the uterus below the pubococcygeal line during straining. Concomitant cystocele.

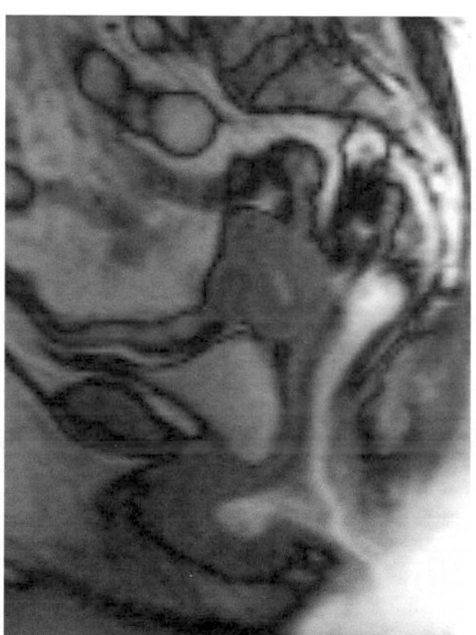

Fig. 4.29 Pelvic organ prolapse with cystocele and rectocele. MRI. Sagittal bSSFP sequence. Bulging of the anterior rectal wall (rectocele) and abnormal descent of the bladder floor (cystocele) during defecation.

- **Course and prognosis**
  Depend on the severity of prolapse • Good in patients with mild prolapse • In severe prolapse, symptoms often persist even after surgical correction.
- **What does the clinician want to know?**
  Severity of prolapse • Which organs are involved?

Differential Diagnosis

Normal mobility of the pelvic organs	– Organs do not descend below the pubococcygeal line
"Physiologic" rectocele	– Rectal bulge of less than 2 cm anterior to the reference line

Tips and Pitfalls

Always perform conventional defecography with opacification of the bladder, small intestine, and vagina so as not to overlook prolapse of these organs • The counter-pressure exerted by a very full bladder masks prolapse because it prevents downward displacement of the uterus.

Selected References

Fletcher JG et al. Magnetic resonance imaging of anatomic and dynamic defects of the pelvic floor in defecatory disorders. Am J Gastroenterol 2003; 98: 399–411

Kelvin FM, Pannu H. Dynamic cystoproctography: fluoroscopic and MRI techniques for evaluating pelvic organ prolapse. In: Bartram CI, DeLancey JOL (eds). Imaging Pelvic Floor Disorders. Heidelberg: Springer; 2003: 51–68

Lienemann A et al. Dynamic MR colpocystorectography assessing pelvic-floor descent. Eur Radiol 1997; 7: 1309–1317

Roos JE et al. Experience of 4 years with open MR defecography: pictorial review of anorectal anatomy and disease. Radiographics 2002; 22: 817–832

Definition

- **Epidemiology**
  Normal follicles are detected in up to 55% of women operated on for ovarian tumors suspected on preoperative ultrasound.
  Ovarian cysts: Larger than typical Graafian follicles during the menstrual cycle (up to 3 cm in diameter) • *Simplest form:* Persisting follicles • May contain blood • *Causes:* Failure of hypothalamic, pituitary, or ovarian regulatory mechanisms • Typically resolve after 2–3 months • Ultrasound follow-up may be indicated after 4–5 months.
  Adjacent cysts, cystic changes: Peritoneal cysts • Paraovarian cysts • Multilocular adhesions after inflammation or surgery • Fluid collections in small cysts of the paroophoron or rete ovarii.
  Polycystic ovaries: Numerous follicular cysts (12 or more) of similar size accumulating under a thickened tunica albuginea • Up to 1 cm in diameter • Anovulation • Bilateral • Typical endocrine symptoms.

Imaging Signs

- **Modality of choice**
  Clinical examination and transvaginal ultrasound • Transvaginal ultrasound for follow-up • Pelvic MRI may be indicated to resolve inconclusive findings.
- **Transvaginal ultrasound findings**
  Usually discovered incidentally at screening • Smoothly delineated, anechoic cystic structures with thin walls • Up to 3 cm in diameter • Follow-up after 4–5 months if no signs of malignancy are present.
- **MRI findings**
  MRI is done with the phased-array body coil after intravenous butylscopolamine • Axial and sagittal T2-weighted images: well-defined, thin-walled cystic structures of high signal intensity • Axial T1-weighted images before and after intravenous contrast administration (e.g., to exclude solid components) • If the cyst content is hyperintense on T1-weighted images, additional fat-saturated T1-weighted sequence to differentiate dermoid cysts (signal decrease with fat saturation) and hemorrhagic cysts (no signal decrease) • *Malignancy criteria:* Solid components (including papillary projections), wall/septum thickness over 3 mm, lesion size over 4 cm (not very reliable).

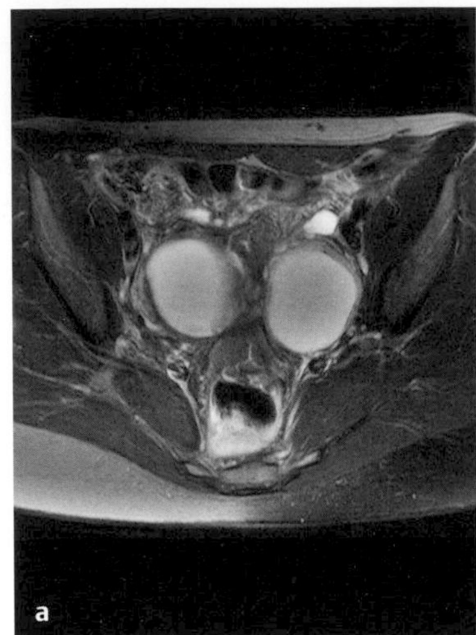

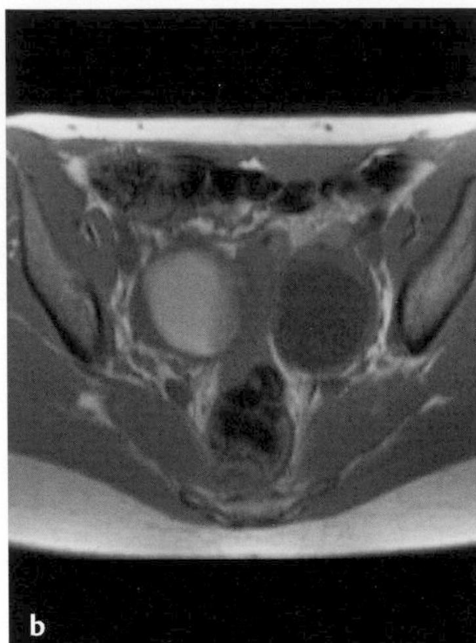

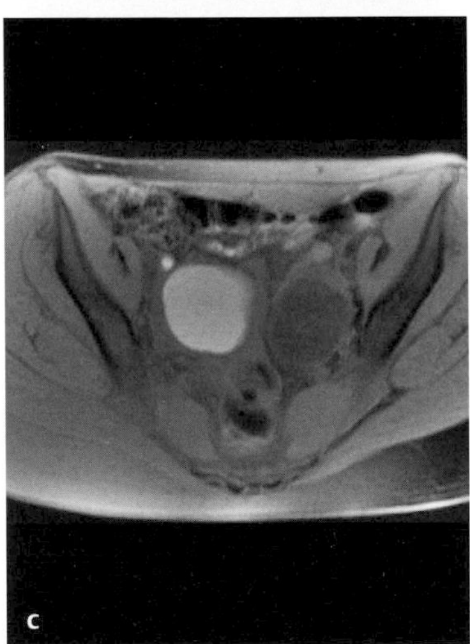

Fig. 4.30 a–c Ovarian cysts.

- **a** Axial T2-weighted MR image. Smooth, thin-walled cysts of both ovaries. No signs of malignancy.
- **b** T1-weighted MR image. High signal intensity of the cyst on the right indicates hemorrhage.
- **c** Fat-saturated T1-weighted MR image. Unchanged high signal intensity of the right cyst excludes a dermoid.

Clinical Aspects

- **Typical presentation**
  Usually asymptomatic.
- **Treatment options**
  Treatment needed only if cysts persist or show signs of malignancy.
- **Course and prognosis**
  Excellent prognosis • Follow-up to exclude malignancy.
- **What does the clinician want to know?**
  Are there signs of malignancy that warrant surgical exploration? • Does the patient have a dermoid cyst or endometriotic cyst ("chocolate cyst")?

Differential Diagnosis

Cystadenoma	– Cystic mass with septa
Cystadenocarcinoma	– Malignancy criteria
Dermoid cyst	– Contains fat

Tips and Pitfalls

Do not biopsy an ovarian tumor.

Selected References

Pfleiderer A. Gutartige Ovarialtumoren und Borderline-Tumoren. Gynäkologe 2002; 35: 689–704

Definition

Accumulation of incompletely developed follicles (more than 12) in the ovaries with thickening of the tunica albuginea • Follicular cysts typically the same size (up to 1 cm) • Ovaries enlarged to over 10 cm^3 • Anovulation • Involves both ovaries • Typical endocrine symptoms including hyperandrogenism, irregular menstrual cycles, and obesity (also known as *Stein–Leventhal syndrome*).

- **Epidemiology**
  Seen in up to 5% of women.
- **Endocrine changes**
  Ovarian granulosa cells do not adequately respond to FSH and LH • The result is increased LH release with subsequent excessive ovarian androgen production.

Imaging Signs

- **Modality of choice**
  Transvaginal ultrasound in women trying to conceive • No other imaging tests needed.
- **Transvaginal ultrasound findings**
  Typically enlargement of both ovaries with a prominent, smooth capsule • Multiple cysts (at least 12) measuring up to 1 cm in diameter • Total ovarian volume increased to over 10 cm^3.
- **MRI and CT findings**
  Same as transvaginal ultrasound • Often incidental finding • Enlarged ovaries containing multiple cysts.

Clinical Aspects

- **Typical presentation**
  Endocrine symptoms: Hyperandrogenism, irregular menstrual cycles, and obesity.
- **Treatment options**
  Depend on severity and whether the woman is trying to conceive • An affected woman who is trying to conceive is treated with metformin, clomifene, gonadotropins, or glucocorticoids • In women not trying to conceive, treatment comprises oral contraceptives and glucocorticoids.
- **Course and prognosis**
  Infertility is common • Increased cardiovascular risk.
- **What does the clinician want to know?**
  Cyst size: less than 1 cm • Ovarian volume • Concomitant genital tract abnormalities.

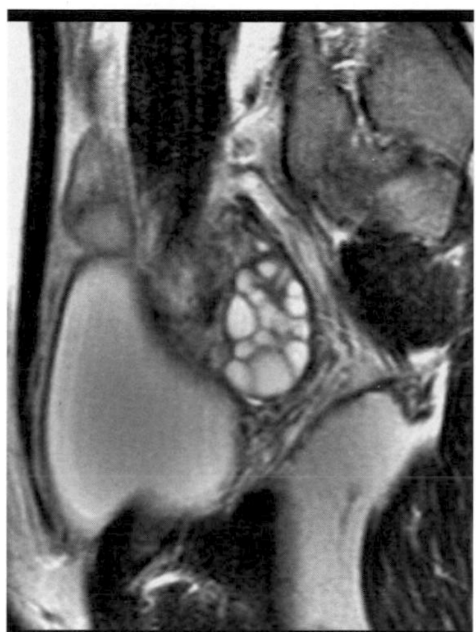

Fig. 4.31 Polycystic ovaries. Sagittal T2-weighted MR image. Good visualization of multiple small cysts.

Differential Diagnosis

Graafian follicles	- At least one cyst over 1 cm - Fewer cysts
Septated cyst	- Typically only one or two septa - Subdivisions not round - Unilateral
Normal variant with multiple small cysts	- In patients without hyperandrogenism and irregular menstrual cycles, polycystic ovarian syndrome is not the first consideration
Cushing disease	- Hormonal constellation - Ovarian findings

Selected References

Balen AH et al. Ultrasound assessment of the polycystic ovary: international consensus definitions. Hum Reprod Update 2003; 9: 505–514

Pfleiderer A. Gutartige Ovarialtumoren und Borderline-Tumoren. Gynäkologe 2002; 35: 689–704

Definition

Neoplasm made up of cells that often contain elements from all three germ layers and can develop into any type of tissue • The majority are benign cystic teratomas (dermoid cysts or mature teratomas) • Contain an oily cystic fluid that may be interspersed with hairs and is surrounded by a firm fibrous capsule • Dermoid plug (Rokitansky protuberance) is typical • Teratomas may contain mature organoid structures such as teeth or ovarian struma • Malignancy is determined by the degree of differentiation of the tissue components.

- **Epidemiology**
  Typically in younger women • Accounts for 20–30% of benign ovarian tumors • Up to 50% in girls.

Imaging Signs

- **Modality of choice**
  Transvaginal ultrasound • CT or MRI to demonstrate fat in teratomas with atypical distribution of tissue elements or a large solid component • Teratomas without fat are virtually impossible to distinguish from malignant ovarian tumors.
- **Transvaginal ultrasound findings**
  Often detected incidentally. Cystic structure with strong capsule. Often fat-fluid interface. Solid portions may contain echogenic structures such as teeth. Ultrasound is not specific for the demonstration of fat.
- **CT findings**
  Often fat-fluid interface with an upper layer of fat attenuation • Enhancing solid components may be present (which are not interpreted as indicating a malignant teratoma if other features strongly suggest a benign tumor) • Teeth may occasionally be demonstrated.
- **MRI findings**
  MRI is performed with a body phased-array coil after intravenous injection of butylscopolamine; axial and sagittal T2-weighted sequences • Liquid components have high signal intensity on T2-weighted images • Fat has high signal on T1-weighted images • Signal drop on fat-saturated T1- or T2-weighted images differentiates fat from hemorrhage • Enhancing solid components may be present • Calcifications appear as signal voids on T1- and T2-weighted images.

Clinical Aspects

- **Typical presentation**
  Often incidental finding in asymptomatic women • Large teratoma may cause sensation of pressure • Sebaceous peritonitis in the rare case of rupture.
- **Treatment options**
  Surgery with excellent prognosis.
- **What does the clinician want to know?**
  Confirmation of the tentative sonographic diagnosis • Signs of malignancy?

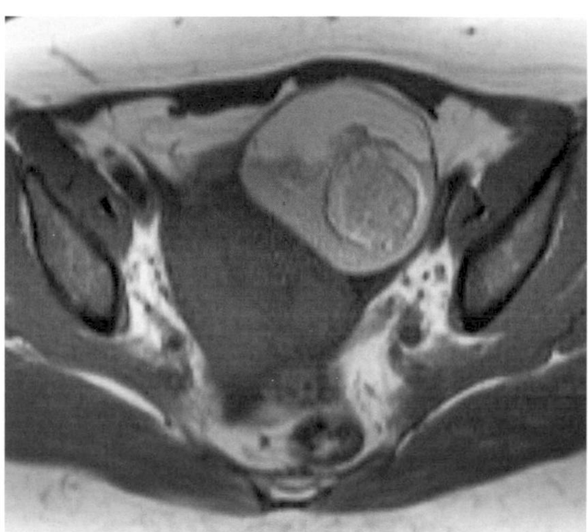

Fig. 4.32 Ovarian teratoma. Axial T1-weighted MR image showing cyst with partially solid contents and layering. Higher signal intensity of upper layer.

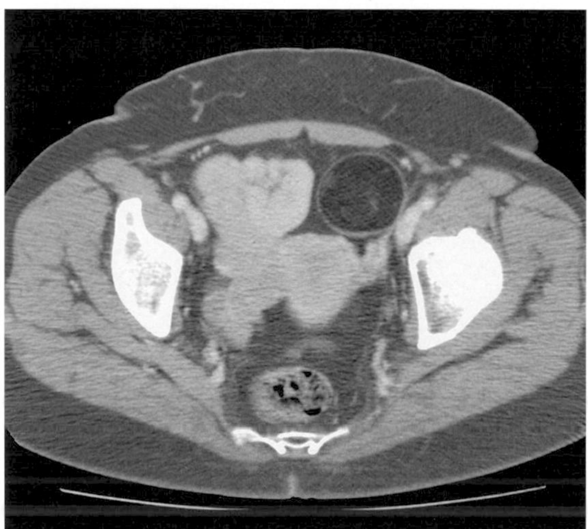

Fig. 4.33 Ovarian teratoma. CT scan showing smooth mass of the left ovary with internal fat attenuation.

Differential Diagnosis

Hemorrhagic cyst	– Unchanged high signal intensity on fat-saturated images
Malignant tumor	– Difficult to differentiate from a purely solid teratoma on CT or MRI unless well-differentiated components such as teeth are present

Tips and Pitfalls

A definitive diagnosis of mature teratoma is difficult to establish unless a signal drop can be demonstrated on fat-saturated images (may otherwise be confused with endometriotic cyst) • Biopsy has been abandoned.

Selected References

Pfleiderer A. Gutartige Ovarialtumoren und Borderline-Tumoren. Gynäkologe 2002; 35: 689–704

Stevens SK et al. Teratomas versus cystic hemorrhagic adnexal lesions: differentiation with proton-selective fat-saturation MR imaging. Radiology 1993; 186: 481–488

Definition

Arise from the superficial ovarian epithelium.
Serous cystadenoma: 20–30% of all benign ovarian tumors • Bilateral in nearly 20% of cases • Contains clear, thin, proteinaceous fluid.
Mucinous cystadenoma: 20% of benign ovarian tumors • Unilateral in 97–98% of cases • Stringy, clear or glassy, gelatinous fluid containing pseudomucin (glycoprotein) • May become very large.

- **Epidemiology**
  Very rare before puberty • 60% of all ovarian tumors.

Imaging Signs

- **Modality of choice**
  Transvaginal ultrasound • Pelvic MRI as a problem-solving tool.
- **Transvaginal ultrasound findings**
  Anechoic, smooth cystic lesion with delicate walls • Diameter over 3 cm • Septa are more common in mucinous cystadenomas • Septa up to 3 mm in thickness.
- **MRI findings**
  MRI is performed with the body phased-array coil after intravenous injection of butylscopolamine; axial and sagittal T2-weighted sequences, axial T1-weighted sequence • Additional T1-weighted sequence after intravenous contrast administration • High signal intensity on T2-weighted images • Smoothly demarcated • Thin walled • Septa may be present • Some variation in intensity between individual locules in mucinous tumors • Malignancy criteria—solid components (including intracystic papillary projections), wall/septum thickness over 3 mm, lesion size over 4 cm (not very reliable).

Clinical Aspects

- **Typical presentation**
  Large cystadenoma can be palpated • Asymptomatic for a long time • Typically an incidental finding at screening • Large tumor is associated with bloating, increased abdominal girth, and symptoms caused by compression of other structures.
- **Treatment options**
  In toto removal • Great care must be taken to avoid intraabdominal rupture.
- **Course and prognosis**
  Mucinous cystadenoma can become very large • Excellent prognosis if complete resection is accomplished • Intraabdominal rupture may produce pseudomyxoma peritonei.
- **What does the clinician want to know?**
  Location • Size • Signs of malignancy?

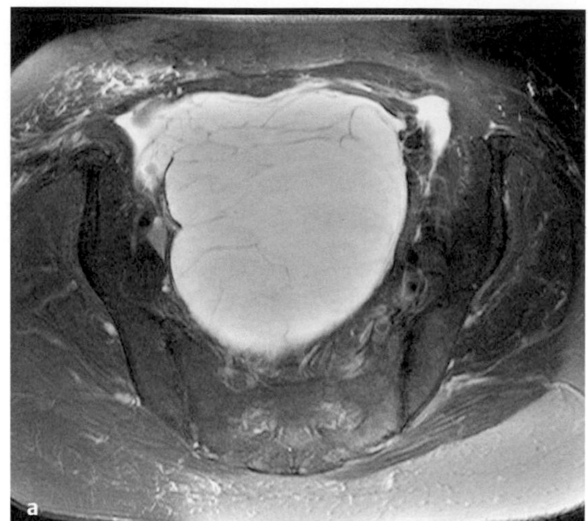

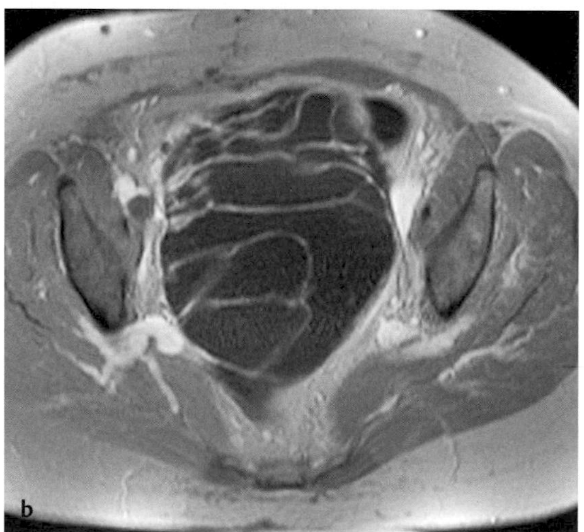

Fig. 4.34 a, b Ovarian cystadenoma. Axial T2-weighted MR image (**a**). Large cyst with septa. No solid components. Axial T1-weighted image after contrast administration (**b**). Enhancement of thin septa.

Differential Diagnosis

Cystadenocarcinoma	– Signs of malignancy – Differentiation may be difficult
Uncomplicated cyst	– No septa – Uniform high signal intensity on T2-weighted images

Tips and Pitfalls

Do not biopsy an ovarian mass • Additional coil elements covering the abdomen are needed for full evaluation of large mucinous cystadenomas which often extend above the umbilical level.

Selected References

Jung SE et al. CT and MR imaging of ovarian tumors with emphasis on differential diagnosis. Radiographics 2002; 22: 1305–1325

Togashi K et al. Ovarian cancer: the clinical role of US, CT and MRI. European Radiology 2003; 13: L78–104

Definition

About 20–30% of all ovarian tumors are malignant • 60–70% of ovarian malignancies are diagnosed when the tumor has already spread within the abdomen • Leading cause of cancer death from gynecologic tumors • Ovarian malignancies arise from epithelial tissue, stroma, or germ cells • Epithelial tumors (carcinomas) account for 70% of cases • Borderline tumors have low malignant potential (histologic features of malignancy but no destructive or infiltrative growth).

Tumor markers: For follow-up • Not a reliable indicator before surgery • CA125 also raised in endometriosis, acute pancreatitis, and uterine adenomyosis • CA72–4 may be determined if CA125 is in the normal range.

- **Staging (FIGO)**
  - I Tumor limited to the ovaries.
    - A Limited to one ovary.
    - B Limited to both ovaries, capsule intact.
    - C Ascites containing malignant cells, capsule ruptured.
  - II Pelvic extension of tumor.
    - A Extension to uterus and/or fallopian tubes.
    - B Extension to other pelvic tissues.
    - C Tumor either IIA or IIB with malignant ascites.
  - III Local tumor spread.
    - A Microscopic seeding of abdominal peritoneal cavity.
    - B Implants ≤ 2 cm of abdominal peritoneal surfaces.
    - C Implants > 2 cm of abdominal peritoneal surfaces or nodal metastases.
  - IV Distant metastases outside the peritoneal cavity.
- **Epidemiology**

  Annual incidence of 16/100 000 women.
- **Risk factors**

  Family history • Increased ovulation rate (e.g., nulliparity).

Imaging Signs

- **Modality of choice**

  Transvaginal ultrasound • MRI.
- **Routine diagnostic workup**

  MRI is superior to CT and ultrasound for tumor characterization.
  - Chest and abdominal CT in patients with signs of ovarian cancer.
  - Colonoscopy and cystoscopy in patients with symptoms of or suspected infiltration • May be supplemented by IVP, abdominal ultrasound.
  - If pleural effusion is present: cytologic test to identify malignant cells (= stage IV disease).
- **Transvaginal ultrasound findings**

  Examination with a 7.5 MHz endoprobe • Good delineation of the ovaries • Good evaluation of cystic structures in most cases • Identification of suspicious solid areas • Presence of ascites.

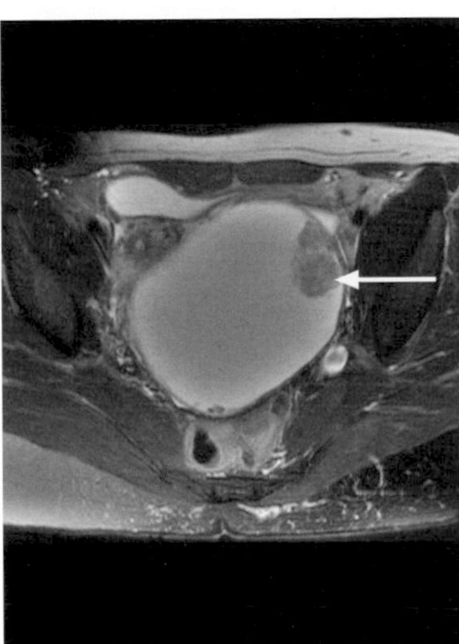

Fig. 4.35 Ovarian carcinoma. Axial T2-weighted MR image showing an ovarian tumor with cystic and solid areas (arrow).

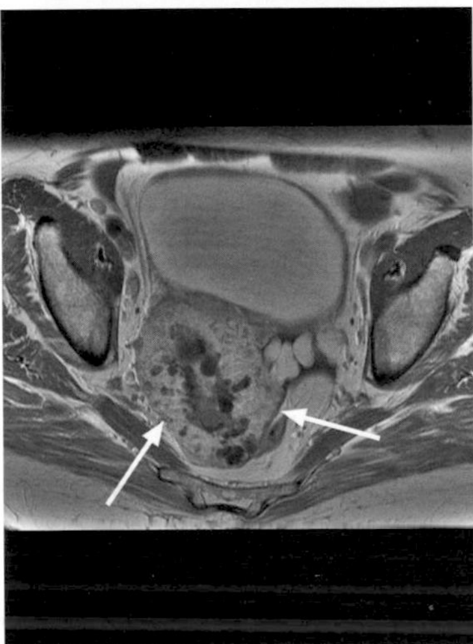

Fig. 4.36 Ovarian carcinoma (arrows). Contrast-enhanced axial T1-weighted MR image. Adenocarcinoma with solid and small cystic areas. Enhancement predominantly of the solid components.

- **CT**
  CT with multiplanar reconstruction • Intravenous and oral contrast medium, additional rectal opacification if needed • Scan range from the diaphragm to the pelvic floor.
- **MRI**
  There is 93% accuracy in tumor characterization • MRI of the pelvis and upper abdomen using a phased-array body coil • T2-weighted TSE sequences in two perpendicular planes and axial T1-weighted sequence • Additional axial PD-weighted sequence covering an area extending above the level of the aortic bifurcation • T1- and T2-weighted sequences of the upper abdomen during breath-hold or with respiratory gating for identification of peritoneal implants • T1-weighted sequence of the upper abdomen and pelvis after contrast administration.
  Malignancy criteria—solid components (including intracystic papillary projections), wall/septum thickness over 3 mm, lesion size over 4 cm (not very reliable).

Clinical Aspects

- **Typical presentation**
  Early stages are asymptomatic • Increased abdominal girth, displacement of adjacent organs, foreign body sensation, and nonspecific pain • Genital bleeding is rare.
- **Treatment options**
  Depend on the tumor stage • Primary surgical management • Hysterectomy, oophorectomy including contralateral ovary, omentectomy, pelvic and paraaortic lymphadenectomy in advanced ovarian cancer • Maximum debulking of very large tumors • Postoperative chemotherapy with carboplatin and paclitaxel.
- **Course and prognosis**
  Advanced ovarian cancer typically associated with massive ascites and distant metastases • 5-year survival rates of 60–90% for stage I to 5% for stage IV.
- **What does the clinician want to know?**
  Malignancy criteria? • Features suggesting benign tumor (e.g., mature teratoma) • Extent of ovarian cancer, especially in terms of peritoneal implants and distant metastases • Lymphadenopathy?

Differential Diagnosis

Cystadenoma	– No solid components; if septa are present, they are very thin
Germ cell tumor	– Cannot be reliable differentiated from ovarian carcinoma
Subserosal leiomyoma	– Relationship to uterus – Low signal intensity on T2-weighted images
Fibroma	– Typically hypointense on T1- and T2-weighted images
Mature teratoma	– Contains fat – May also have solid components

Tips and Pitfalls

Diagnostic puncture of ovarian tumors has been abandoned • Care must be taken to differentiate metastases of the liver capsule (stage IIIB) from intrahepatic metastases (stage IV).

Selected References

Forstner R. CT and MRI in ovarian carcinoma. In: Hamm B, Forstner R (eds). MRI and CT of the female pelvis. Heidelberg: Springer; 2006

Togashi K. Ovarian cancer: the clinical role of US, CT and MRI. Eur Radiol 2003; 13: 87–104

Yamashita Y et al. Adnexal masses: Accuracy of characterization with transvaginal US and precontrast and postcontrast MR imaging. Radiology 1995; 194: 557–565

Definition

About 4% of all ovarian tumors • Arise from the nonspecialized mesenchymal ovarian stroma • Fibroma must be differentiated from fibrosarcoma • Ascites is present in 10% of patients with ovarian fibroma and hydrothorax in 1%, especially with tumors over 10 cm in size (Meigs syndrome).

- **Epidemiology**
  Ovarian fibromas occur at any age but are more common in women over 50. Typically unilateral.

Imaging Signs

- **Modality of choice**
  Transvaginal ultrasound for screening • MRI for tumor characterization.
- **Transvaginal ultrasound findings**
  Ultrasound is performed with a 7.5 MHz endoprobe • Good delineation of the ovaries • Good evaluation of cystic components in most cases • Solid tumor • Little or no growth over time.
- **MRI findings**
  MRI has 93% accuracy in tumor characterization • Solid lesion of low signal intensity on T1- and T2-weighted images • Slight to marked contrast enhancement.
- **CT findings**
  CT with multiplanar reconstruction capabilities in patients with suspected ovarian tumor • Precontrast examination • Postcontrast examination after intravenous and oral contrast administration with additional rectal opacification if needed • Scan range from the diaphragm to the pelvic floor • Solid, well-defined tumor in most cases • No or only small cystic component • CT does not allow reliable differentiation from malignant tumors.

Clinical Aspects

- **Typical presentation**
  Asymptomatic • Often diagnosed in women undergoing cancer screening.
- **Treatment options**
  Resection or follow-up.
- **Course and prognosis**
  Excellent prognosis.
- **What does the clinician want to know?**
  Signs of malignancy? • Specific diagnosis if possible.

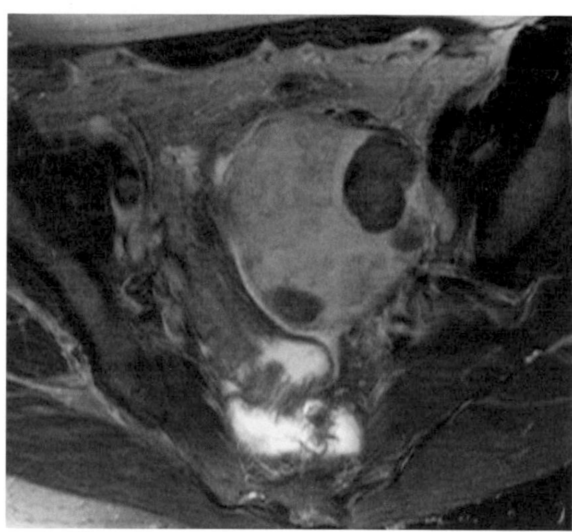

Fig. 4.37 Ovarian fibroma. Axial T2-weighted MR image showing an ovarian mass with hypointense areas.

Differential Diagnosis

Granulosa-theca cell tumor	- Similar in morphologic appearance, estrogen-producing sex cord stromal tumor - Rare, typically occurs after menopause
Ovarian malignancy, e.g., fibrosarcoma	- Inhomogeneous composition - At times difficult to separate from fibroma

Tips and Pitfalls

Do not biopsy an ovarian mass.

Selected References

Outwater EK et al. Ovarian fibromas and cystadenofibromas: MRI features of the fibrous component. J Magn Res Imaging 1997; 7: 465–471

Yamashita Y et al. Adnexal masses: Accuracy of characterization with transvaginal US and precontrast and postcontrast MR imaging. Radiology 1995; 194: 557–565

A

B

C

Page numbers in *italics* refer to illustrations.

D

E

I

K

L

M

N

O

V